Your
Heart
and You

Other books by Elizabeth Wilde McCormick

The Heart Attack Recovery Book
Surviving Breakdown
Change for the Better
Healing the Heart
Living on the Edge
Transpersonal Psychotherapy, Theory and Practice (with Nigel
   Wellings)

Your Heart and You

A HOLISTIC GUIDE TO A HEALTHIER HEART

Elizabeth Wilde McCormick
and Dr Leisa Freeman

PIATKUS

Copyright © 2001 Elizabeth Wilde McCormick
and Dr Leisa Freeman

First published in 2002 by
Judy Piatkus (Publishers) Limited
5 Windmill Street
London W1T 2JA
e-mail: info@piatkus.co.uk

The moral right of the authors has been asserted

A catalogue record for this book is available from the British Library

ISBN 0 7499 2203 6

Edited by Lizzie Hutchins
Text design by Paul Saunders

This book has been printed on paper manufactured with respect for the
environment using wood from managed sustainable resources

Typeset by Action Publishing Technology Ltd, Gloucester
Printed and bound in Great Britain by
Biddles Ltd, Guildford & King's Lynn
www.biddles.co.uk

This book is dedicated to John Stanley McCormick

NOVEMBER 1924–MAY 1999

CONTENTS

PART 4 *Recovery and Rehabilitation*

PART 5 *Keeping Your Heart Healthy*

PREFACE

by Elizabeth McCormick

I have worked as a psychological counsellor and psychotherapist in many settings since 1979 and have been writing books since before this time. In the last 15 years I have also been workshop leader, psychotherapy and supervision trainer and teacher. I am currently a consultant to the Centre for Transpersonal Psychology in London, and a supervision and training tutor in Cognitive Analytic Therapy (short-term therapy) at Guy's Hospital, also in London.

I first became interested in the heart when my husband John had a heart attack in August 1977 while on holiday in Trinidad. A 60-cigarette-a-day smoker, a busy man running his own company who, in his own words, 'thrived on stress', he had to make huge changes. So did our large extended family as we sought to support him in regaining his health.

My first book about the heart, *The Heart Attack Recovery Book*, published in 1984 and reissued in 1989, was the result of my own experience and research into the emotional and psychological issues following a heart attack, issues that busy doctors frequently have little time to address. John's own doctor's instruction – 'Go home and relax' – had no fertile ground in which to grow. Relaxing was alien to him and at the same time he was much too angry with his body for letting him down to accept something as 'weedy' as relaxation. I have discovered this is a common response at first. Heart patients need time to digest the experience and a plan for what they might do with their emotional frustration before they can make use of a rehabilitation programme, of which there are now many.

While working as a psychological counsellor in the cardiac department of Charing Cross Hospital in 1984 I met Dr Leisa Freeman, who was working as a cardiologist there and was regarded as something of a legend.

My second book on the heart, *Healing the Heart*, was published in 1993 and looked at the interrelationship between the physical heart, 'the worker heart', and the heart of the emotions, 'the feeling heart'. By this time John had had a coronary artery bypass operation and a new lease of life. I had developed further my interest in issues of the heart. My prime concern as a psychologist and meditation practitioner is: what do we do with emotion?

This book was commissioned in 1999, just after John's heart condition had begun deteriorating – he had been fitted with a pacemaker after a third-degree heart block – and while he was waiting for more cardiac surgery.

Very sadly, he died at Papworth Hospital in May 1999 after complications following his second bypass operation. He was a big man, wonderful, funny, generous and brave, who, despite 22 years of heart disease, lived his life to the very full. We had always shared his journey of the heart and he was keen that I should offer whatever could be helpful to other people. He was also deeply fond of my co-author Dr Leisa Freeman, who helped us through John's last year of ill health.

Leisa and I write this book with a full heart and in memory of him.

by Dr Leisa Freeman

Following training in medicine at the University of Birmingham Medical School and a pre-registration year in Birmingham and Barnet, I completed an SHO rotation in general medicine at University College Hospital, London. I was a registrar in cardiology and general medicine at Charing Cross Hospital, London, and then spent time in research. The main area of my research was the effect of psychological stress on patients with different types of heart disease. I have published most of my research in medical journals and written chapters on emotion and the heart in medical textbooks: *Diseases of the Heart* (Balliere and Tindall, 1989) and *Difficult Cardiology 111*, 1997. I then continued my training at the National Heart Hospital and now work as a cardiologist at the Norfolk and Norwich Hospital, where I have a particular interest in adults born with congenital heart disease.

As doctors, while most of us appreciate the effect of emotion on the heart, which can be quite profound in some cases, we do not always have the resources and time to direct people to help themselves or to suggest other allied professionals who can provide guidance over and above the medication or interventions we suggest. This can be frustrating. When I met Elizabeth McCormick at Charing Cross Hospital, she and other therapists there demonstrated the resources and skills that are available. It was therefore a great pleasure to be asked to join Elizabeth in writing this book.

ACKNOWLEDGEMENTS

Many people have contributed to the thinking and presentation of this book. The authors would like to thank their respective patient spouses, David Cargill and John McCormick, for their support and patience during the time-consuming process of creation.

Many thanks go to the editorial staff at Piatkus Books – Gill, Kate, Sandra, Ann and in particular Lizzie Hutchins for their considerable labours on behalf of the book structure.

Thanks to Mark Dunn for permission to use the poem on page 242 from his private collection. Quotations from the film *The Heart Has Its Reasons*, directed by Mark Kidel and shown on Channel 4.

Elizabeth McCormick would like to make a personal thanks to the intensive care nurses at Papworth Hospital, from whom she learned a great deal about the care of the heart in all aspects. John Walwick and John Dunning, cardiothoracic surgeons at Papworth Hospital who looked after John McCormick, also gave their time to discuss matters related to the heart for the purposes of this book.

Deep thanks go to Thich Nhat Hanh for his worldwide teachings on the mindfulness practices in daily life and the deep listening with an informed heart. I (Elizabeth) give thanks to my colleagues Susie Nixon, and Moira MacLean, who contributed directly to the text in Chapter 15. Many thanks for the generosity of all those who kindly gave taped interviews about their personal experience of living with heart disease – Mark Price and his daughter Esther, Betty and Margaret, and to those providing all the other stories where names have been changed to protect identity.

Lastly I offer gratitude to my friends and colleagues and my co-author Leisa Freeman, who supported me throughout the long creation of this book, through my husband John's death in the middle of writing it and in the demanding process of coming back to it one year later. They also read and commented upon the final drafts: Ann Shearer, Phillippa Vick, Claire Chappell, Gill Wilson, Nigel Wellings.

INTRODUCTION

Physical heart disease may be the final manifestation of
years of abuse that begins in the psyche and spirit....
Heart disease is a metaphor as well as an anatomical illness.

DEAN ORNISH, American cardiologist

THE HEART IS the most potent organ in the body for most
people. How we relate to our heart, whether in a physical
or emotional sense, makes a difference to its care, and ultimately to its lifecycle.

This book addresses the understanding and care of the
heart as a central physical organ as well as the heart of our
poetic imaginations – the emotional, 'feeling' heart. It explores
how the two are linked, why understanding this link is important and how we might build a bridge between the two.
Coming from two different but complementary professional
disciplines – psychotherapy and cardiology – we have woven
our clinical knowledge and experience together in support of
this bridge.

Heart disease has reached epidemic proportions in
Western industrialised nations for both men and women.
There are 175,000 deaths from heart disease per year in the
UK, with thousands more suffering heart failure, at a cost of
£1.6 billion, and it is estimated that 75 per cent of people go to

their doctor with problems that are connected to stress and to feeling 'sick at heart'.

There are many world-wide research projects and studies that have concentrated upon finding causes for heart disease and this book will refer to several of them. Primarily, though, we concentrate upon helping you to help yourself.

The book explores the following areas:

♦ Helping you to understand the links between stress, emotions and your heart.

♦ Empowering you to take charge of the care of your heart in the ways most suited to your personality and emotional need.

♦ Getting across accurate medical information so that you can gain the confidence to make informed decisions.

♦ Demystifying and detoxifying some of the powerful and unhelpful myths that surround heart problems.

♦ Sharing stories from heart patients so that you can relate to their experiences.

The book begins by looking at emotions and your heart as this is an area that has long been neglected by both the medical profession and patients alike, but which is, we believe, absolutely crucial to maintaining health. Biomolecular scientists now suggest that all living systems are by their nature systems of energy that contain information about what they are and how they function. From psychoneuroimmunology – the psychological science that studies the relationship between the brain, the immune system and the experience of the outside world – comes the information that nothing is ever lost, that human cells have receptors, even 'wisdom' and memory, that consciousness precedes matter. Examples of this understanding come from the work of Professor Paul Pearsall in his book *The Heart's Code* and Dr Candace Pert in her book *Molecules of Emotion* and Jacques Benveniste in *The Memory of Water*.

These findings encourage us to take responsibility for the way in which we live in our bodies. They suggest that our attitude and beliefs *can* make a difference. This becomes crucial when our physical heart suffers from blocked arteries, from the demands of high blood pressure, from the pain of angina. For the heart is the most central system of all, with its ever-busy pumping action responsible for the transmission of millions of blood cells around the body all the time. The heart does enough work in terms of effort in one day to raise a ton weight to the height of a five-storey building. It is the strongest muscle in the body and the most sensitive. When it 'speaks', this may be the signal we've been unconsciously waiting for in order to open up emotionally and psychologically.

Each of us can learn to listen to our own heart. We only have to accept that our heart acts as both a central organ for the regulation of blood and oxygen, and as a wise 'feeling intelligence' that can guide us on our way.

For many people, it is the physical heart that 'speaks' first, bringing them into intimate contact with their feelings, many of which they did not realise they had. You may have had a heart attack, for example, or suffered chest pain that led to investigations for heart disease, or perhaps suffered symptoms that led to you discovering you had raised blood pressure.

When the heart speaks physically we have to learn to take care of it. This always means making changes – changes in diet, exercise, work and rest. It means an adjustment in your response to life because life can no longer be taken for granted. Mortality has beckoned. As a result you may feel fear, anger, resentment, anxiety, loss and a desire to sort out old and current life issues. You may find you have the desire to make use of the gift of time in the best possible way – what many people, including my husband John (McCormick), call 'living on borrowed time'.

Alternatively, it may be that you have not been diagnosed with a heart problem, but you simply know in your heart that something is wrong with your body and act upon it. You may not trust your instinct, because it is not scientific and you are afraid of being ridiculed, or you cannot face doing anything about it. But it is becoming increasingly evident from research – and from our own clinical practice – that you should really listen to what you know in your heart.

Part 1 of this book, therefore, focuses on helping you to understand this fundamental link between body and mind.

Chapter 1 explains the connection between feelings, emotions and the physical heart. It shows how the heart becomes stressed if we are unable to cope with difficult feelings and demands, and offers exercises designed to recognise and help this situation.

While the word 'stress' is widely used today and the links between body and mind are more recognised, many of us do not really understand stress, how it emerges in our life or what to do about it. Often, we are stressed just knowing we are stressed! In Chapter 2 you will find more about the role of stress and how you can learn to cope with it.

Part 2 looks in detail at your physical heart. It begins in Chapter 3 by describing the functions of the heart and the various components of the heart so that you can better understand what happens when things go wrong, and to get you familiar with medical terminology.

If you have recently been diagnosed with a problem relating to your heart you may want to know more about your specific condition. Chapters 4, 5, 6 and 7 look at different heart problems, the associated risk factors and what you can do. Chapter 8, 'Cardiac Tests and Monitoring', will help you understand the procedures that may have been recommended in the way of treatment.

In Part 3 we look at the differences between the male and female heart, and the different health issues relating to each.

Part 4 looks principally at recovery and rehabilitation. If you have had a heart attack, a bypass or valve repair operation and are wondering how to cope with rehabilitation, Chapters 12, 13 and 14 attempt to address many of the everyday issues that emerge during these times, including what happens during cardiac surgery and how to manage your time in intensive care and aftercare at home.

In Part 5 we give you strategies to maintain good health, from diet and exercise tips to recommended complementary therapies.

How to Use This Book

This book will be of benefit to all heart patients, whatever their diagnosis, to people who have a family history of heart disease, to people concerned about how to look after their heart and to partners, spouses or friends of a heart patient. It is designed so that you may select the area that most concerns you about your heart and begin from this point. You don't have to read everything, just the parts that support your own choice of programme of health or that of your partner, friend or member of your family.

Bear in mind that it is all very well being given information about rehabilitation, exercise and diet, but it stays in the abstract until we act upon it and bring it into our lives. How we do this involves learning to look after ourselves in new ways. Because emotions affect the heart, ways in which we may name and understand emotion and what we do with emotion are central aspects of the self-help offered within this book.

If you are reading this book in order to understand what is happening to a partner or friend, you will find that each chapter is complete in itself and as far as possible is written in simple jargon-free language. You may also do the exercises if you wish. Any understanding and communication you are able to achieve will benefit your loved one and reduce the fear that comes from lack of information.

Your Heart and You aims to be a fully comprehensive book about all heart problems that approaches the heart in a holistic, compassionate way, aiming to link you with your heart, mind, body, feelings and spirit.

PART ONE

Understanding the Emotional Heart

Chapter 1

THE FEELING HEART

Give me that man
that is not passion's slave and I will wear him
in my heart's core, ay, in my heart of heart.
WILLIAM SHAKESPEARE, *Hamlet*

THIS CHAPTER IS devoted to the heart that is not seen when surgeons open the chest. Here, the word 'heart' is a shorthand for a variety of our individual expressions, those senses, feelings, intuitions and metaphors that express our innermost being. So as well as a physical heart we have an invisible 'feeling' heart that resonates inside us all the time and links us to our experiences and the deeper core of our being. This heart, with its poetic language, takes us directly into our intimate inner life, our psychology, our hopes, fears and aspirations.

Our attitudes and struggles within this feeling heart have implications for our physical heart. Research has shown that long-term anxiety and depression contribute to heart disease, as do long-buried anger and hostility. Both these emotions stimulate the hormones noradrenaline and cortisol which, when produced without relief or control, are harmful to the heart and circulation.

The heart and circulation respond similarly to pain, fear,

anger and rage. The anticipation of pain or pleasure, a sudden shift in rules or the order of things, or the failure of usual coping strategies also produce circulatory changes. The heart and breathing rate, blood pressure and the forcefulness of the heartbeat all increase in preparation for fight or flight. It is only when these physical responses are not relieved that the situation becomes potentially harmful. So, if your heart is darkened by anger, enraged with hostility or has closed its muscular fist in anger at the world, it is more prone to disease. It is important, therefore, that you get to know your feeling heart and the way it 'speaks' to you, so that you can be in friendship with it and not live in fear of it or shut it down.

Getting in Touch with the Feeling Heart

We may know something, in the head, for forty years. But it is not until it has touched us in the heart that we really take notice of it.

CARL JUNG

The feeling heart makes itself known to us all of the time but we are not always able to receive its messages. This may be because we have not learned how to listen to it or we have shut it down for a while. During times of extreme stress, it can feel just too vulnerable to contact. It may be that in your early life you had to protect yourself from any feeling at all, because no one was there for you or feelings were denied or despised. As a result of this, many of your later activities may be taking place without a feeling connection. You may move into harsh or abusive relationships or take on excessive work tasks because you are unable to feel what is harmful or nourishing for you. Both these experiences will create stress as well as pain and loneliness. Being out of touch with the feeling heart can be at the root of chronic stress.

Many people are afraid of feeling anything at all. This fear is usually because of the emotion that has gathered around what began as a simple feeling. For example, feeling angry we may have unconsciously gathered lots of associations and ideas that have attached themselves to the anger. We may assume 'If I'm angry then I am bad and will be rejected' or 'If I'm angry I will get out of control and no one will be there for me.' So added to the feeling of anger is an entire emotional world of rage, frustration, fear, sadness and loss. Too often, feeling is seen as negative because the emotions created around it feel overwhelming. Anxiety, anger, envy and sadness may feel frightening just because of the energy surrounding them, so also the emotions surrounding loss, bereavement, abandonment and betrayal.

Feeling itself is basically *information*. It is our ideas about this information that tend to give us stress. For example, loss is thought to be always 'bad', but it may mean creating freedom for something new to come into your life.

> Feeling is the vehicle through which life has value.

Feeling is the energy which brings us to an understanding of the value of our experiences. All feeling is valuable – it tells us we are alive. Once you can identify a feeling and then begin to understand all you construct around that feeling, you are in a better position to make authentic connections with the entire range of your feelings and not let them become an emotional burden. When feeling and thinking, head and heart, are no longer either fused together or split apart by fear, they may come together harmoniously, allowing us to use these capacities creatively.

Dr Dean Ornish, author of *Reversing Heart Disease*, who runs a clinic in California devoted to helping patients recover from heart disease, writes of the overwhelming sense of isolation in his heart groups, where patients have expressed being 'isolated from their own feelings, from other people and from something spiritual'. In the safe space of the groups they have been helped to begin sharing feelings about their lives safely.

Finding a safe way to develop words for our feelings means that we are helping to connect with the truth of what we carry inside our heartspace and to choose what we bring out into the outside world.

The most important point about connecting with feeling is that it connects us individually to ourselves and how we are at any time of the day or night. Many heart patients are afraid that feeling will damage their heart or exacerbate their symptoms. Catharsis for the sake of it which is not connected to a true flow of feeling is not necessary. But after a serious illness many people do experience a powerful flow of feeling (*see William, page 18, and Betty, page 174*), which is a release and serves to connect us with our inner reality, about which we can then take some action.

Once you have decided that you are going to build the bridge into your feeling life, there are very clear, safe and well-trodden steps you can take.

Building a Bridge to Your Feelings

♦ Acknowledge that what is happening to you – perhaps through your body feeling down, sick, tense or heavy – may be the expression of a feeling.

♦ Stay with it for a while in whatever form it has emerged. Don't try to do anything to make sense of it. Just offer a kind acceptance.

♦ See if any words come to you that will name and describe it.

♦ Keep staying with the feeling and see if it tells you where it wants to go or what it needs, or if it is a relief just to be recognised.

Once you can acknowledge and name your feelings you are in a position to make a choice about them. Feeling sad, you may express feeling by tears or by asking a kind friend to hold your hand. Feeling angry, you can learn to respect your anger and let the storm of anger rage through you. Feeling happy, you may decide to dance, sing, make music, walk in the countryside or share your joy with others.

Feelings do not stay fixed in one place even though we sometimes feel stuck. Think of the language you might use to describe what you feel – being in a box, in mud, in a deep pool or even an ocean wave, particularly at times of transition or loss. If you are in conscious relationship with your feelings through your bridge-building process, your awareness gives you power and control. You may choose simply to acknowledge that you have a certain feeling. You may surrender to that feeling. Also – and this is important to your freedom – you may choose *not* to explore feeling.

Thinking and Feeling with Your Heart

When we use our heart as the centre for both thinking and feeling, we move the energy of our consciousness down into the area of the chest that involves the function of the lungs, diaphragm, oesophagus, neck, shoulders, arms and the heart itself – what I call the 'heartspace'. Try this for yourself and notice the difference energetically between thinking and feeling from the heart and from the head.

Head and Heart

When we move the focus of our energy and attention away from the head area and down into the heart, we have to slow down. This involves becoming more aware of our breathing. Often the nature of your breathing tells you a lot about how you really feel. This is particularly important because feelings such as anger and hostility are known to play a part in heart problems.

Only when you get close to feeling can you do anything about it. So getting close to the chest and the breath will help you be open to receive messages from the heart. In the heart area we may slow our breathing and relax the surrounding muscles of the neck, shoulders and the abdomen. When we have rested in this way, we are ready to listen to the heart.

When we function from our head only, we tend to develop fixed thoughts and ideas, and can get stuck in the illusion that control is all that matters. We may begin to believe that we can sort everything out through will and determination, through our own ego. When all our energy is given over to this way of functioning, we lose sight of our being as a whole. We tend to lose touch with what we feel, with the more unconscious expressions such as in dream language, in spontaneous images and in our imagination. We may even begin to be afraid of what we feel and of our intuition, because the more we try to control everything with our thinking, the more the unexpressed aspects of ourselves will protest, sometimes even in the form of an accident or heart attack.

Whether our heart problems seem to be a result of our genetic predisposition or a response to stress or living 'lop-sidedly', we do need to listen to both our head and our heart in order to understand ourselves, and to achieve healthy balance.

The Heartspace

Many of the experiences of being human involve the heart-space. What we bring to the heartspace and the way in which we come to use it is governed by the person we are and the lifestyle we choose, and these two are in turn governed by the attitudes, presumptions and coping strategies learned from our parents and teachers.

The heartspace can bring forth many different images and metaphors and we can learn to listen to what it is telling us and become aware of what that means for us. We all use the expression 'heartache', for example, but we rarely explore its actuality. The heart itself and the heartspace can feel heavy after loss and disappointment – this is the leaden heart of despair, the broken heart of bereavement. Your heart can be 'in your boots' and you might not 'have the heart' for anything. Our language gives us the many poetic descriptions of how a heart can feel – the soaring heart of the songbird, the black heart of rage and revenge, the apprehensive 'heart in the mouth', the impervious heart of stone, the cold heart of indifference. Our personal truth lies in our 'heart of hearts'. Our conscience often rests within our heart. Our heart can 'bleed' for another. We have a 'heart to heart'; we speak 'from the heart'; we 'warm the cockles of our heart'. These are the everyday expressions which convey some vivid personal truth about what is happening within our heartspace.

It is important to understand the nature of our heartspace and the ways in which we habitually use it and to be able to 'read' it, because this is where many of our difficulties are first evident.

ALLAN

Allan, who went to hospital suffering from acute chest pain, found relief from talking about his fear of dying from a sudden heart attack as his father had done at the age of 33, the age of Allan's next birthday. The fear itself had led to chronic hyperventilation, to avoidance of going out in case something happened, to isolation and panic attacks. The process of naming the fear, 'getting it off his chest', helped Allan to understand how the chest pain came about. At the same time he learned to practise breathing techniques to help manage his anxiety. He got a dog and started to take steps into the outside world and to find situations where he could talk to other people and thus reduce his isolation. His chest pain diminished and he started learning about how to take care of his heart properly.

Many people are afraid to discover what they really feel, or think, as if conscious awareness will be worse than ignorance. But we have learned in our work with heart patients and in psychotherapy that while painful feelings may be anticipated with fear, once released, there is a freedom from fear, a lightness of being.

To 'get things off your chest' is to create more space for contemplation upon what is most important now. It also can involve a shared understanding with another person, the 'heart to heart' the heart longs for. Therapists, physicians, surgeons and healers who work in contemplative practice all train themselves to listen with every part of their being, with body, mind, heart and soul, so that they become skilled in this art of heart communication. You can learn these skills, too, to help you understand your heart and take better care of it.

Getting in Touch with Your Heart

The following exercises are designed to help you get in touch with your own heart. Knowing what your heart is feeling and carrying helps you to lessen its burden and to take action to relieve its suffering.

● WORD ASSOCIATION

Write the word 'heart' in a circle.

Time yourself for just one minute and write around the circle all your associations with the word.

Just ponder on these words and the feeling in them. 'Feel into' the different stories behind any of the words and allow this to become information. Throughout this book you will be gathering information about how you use the effort of your heart and the heartspace around it.

● TALK TO YOUR HEART

Try sitting down comfortably, dropping your shoulders, concentrating on slow regular in-breaths and slightly longer out-breaths, and then put your hand on your heart and talk to it. Prompt it to reply as you would a close friend. Ask open questions, for example:

● How are you?

● How long have you felt like this?

● What do you most long for?

● What/who can most help you now?

● Is there anything you wish to say?

Listen to all the answers you receive without judgement but with kindness. Write the answers in a notebook so that you can refer back to them later on.

Imagination and the Heart

Another way of communicating with the feeling heart is through our imagination in visualisation and imaging exercises. We may also get in touch with our heart through concentrated silence, as in meditative and contemplative practice. Allowing your imagination to link you with your inner landscape is one way to learn what you need to know about your feeling heart.

When I (Elizabeth) work with heart patients I often ask what their heart means to them. Sometimes people shrug and look puzzled and say, 'It's just a bit of muscle, isn't it?' Sometimes, after a pause, someone will say, 'My heart brings me back to what's going on,' or 'I've been heavy-hearted since Mum died' or even 'I know my heart is worn out.' These responses show that just under the surface of our awareness we have a symbolic imaginative language that we can use to connect directly with our feeling heart.

Some people unconsciously put their hand on the hearts while speaking. If asked what they are feeling under their hand, they may say, 'My heart is full,' or 'There's a hole in my heart right now.' This may be the beginning of an exploration of the feeling heart.

Telephone Line to the Heart

When we have developed an imaginative language with which to explore our heart and our heartspace, we have a telephone line to our heart. We can use this line to give our heart the help it needs to recover after a crisis such as angina or heart attack, and after surgery. We can use it to keep well. By keeping an open telephone line, we are more likely to be aware of the stresses upon the heartspace and what measures need to be taken to strengthen ourselves. By keeping in touch with both what we are feeling and what that feeling most needs, we will be serving our heart both emotionally and physically.

CONNECTING A TELEPHONE LINE TO YOUR HEART

- Sit quietly, with your hand on your heart, and breathe gently.

- As you breathe in, become aware of your heart.

- As you breathe out, relax into the heart.

- Continue breathing in and out in this way for a few minutes.

- Become aware of any feeling, image, colour shape or word that emerges when you ask: 'What is happening in my heart right now?'

- You might like to stop at this point and simply sit with the feeling or follow it wherever it wants to go, or you might find an image appearing, the image of water, fire, a tree, a knot, a mangled engine, a weeping willow. You might get a memory, someone's voice saying something.

- Just stay with whatever comes. Do not judge it. If it is an image, notice everything you can about it – colour, shape, quality, atmosphere.

- You may like to write down or draw what came to you.

- Spend a few minutes contemplating the feeling content of whatever came to you through your telephone link and ponder on it. Let the information just seep into your being. If the exercise has given you a helpful idea or message, you might consider how you would bring this into your life.

WILLIAM (*See also page 164*)

I thought doing the questionnaire I was sent by you for the book was going to be very difficult, but it turned out to be helpful. I had two quite different images of the heart. One was the idea of a mechanical pump ticking away doing the job of a life-support system, coping with whatever life demands. I was breathing and concentrating as I was trying to meditate on the heart, and I had this feeling of slow movement in harmony with breathing, and that if one breathes slowly and steadily it calms the heart and is life-sustaining. So my second image was of the sea, of a calmness and strength like the sea when it is not at all agitated, just gently swelling and subsiding. This made me think of the long-term enduring capability of the heart, in contrast to the pump, which is precise activity. It can just be there sustaining life, without any kind of pressure. I feel it will look after me. If I can have this time when I just let the heart be, it will carry me along calmly and everything will fall into place.

Responding to Emotion

If someone comes along and shoots an arrow into your heart,
it's fruitless to stand there and yell at the person. Much better
to turn your attention to the fact that there's an arrow in your
heart and to relate to that wound.

PEMA CHODRON, *Start Where You Are*

Once we have connected our telephone line to the heart, the
next step is to allow the feeling itself to be fully present for us.
This means living in the present moment and being truly
present, without judgement, with our experience. It means
giving everything our full attention. When we see a beautiful
sunset or the blossoming of a flower, the smile of a friend, a
letter from a lover, we are present with our feelings of happiness. If someone is giving us a hard time, we are present with
the hard time. When we are grief-stricken, we are fully present
with the reality of the broken heart.

The Vietnamese Zen Buddhist Master Thich Nhat Hanh
invites us to imagine ourselves as a tree with roots, a firm
trunk and branches, which is sometimes heavy with blossom.
The tree must face many different kinds of weather, just as we
must face storms in our emotional life.

Thich Nhat Hanh tells of the monk who went out one fine
day into the woods and left the windows of his house open to
allow the breeze to ventilate his rooms. When he returned a
high wind had entered the house and blown all the papers
from his desk into disarray. He uses this story to illustrate how
this process can happen within ourselves. If all our energy is
tied up in our heads or we are whirling around in 'hurry sickness' trying to will ourselves to get things done, the high wind
will get tangled up in our branches and our tree will be in
danger. If, however, we have learned to strengthen the trunk of
the tree and stretch energy into the deep roots, our tree will be
able to withstand the wind.

The practice called mindfulness (*see pages 213–16*) helps us
to focus on the present moment. We are mindful of our breath,

of our feelings, of our feet as we walk, of the food that we are placing in our mouth. This strengthens our ability to be in the present moment. It means we strengthen the trunk of the tree so that when the storms and high winds come we are prepared because all our energy is not in our branches. By training ourselves in the 'little rains' of the everyday, we will be ready for any storm.

Through mindfulness of feeling we can develop a greater fluidity towards our feelings – even feelings such as fear, anxiety and sadness – so that we flow with the feeling rather than having to fight it off. This means that we are less likely to become stressed by the emotions around feeling and to compromise our heart.

Mindfulness of breathing and of feeling (*see exercises in Chapter 16*) also helps expand our everyday awareness into our spiritual nature. Spirituality is not elsewhere, it is where we are in the here and now. It is in the everyday connections with others and the universe. It is in the sense of ourselves as being more than the sum total of our everyday selves or our suffering. Spirituality is not limited to organised religious doctrine or dogma. Connecting to a spiritual dimension and living with this energy helps us to be less dominated by our attachments to a material world or by a need to keep running into the future. It means that we create a spaciousness within ourselves. This alone can be deeply nurturing.

The Emotions of the Broken Heart

The metaphor of the broken heart is familiar to all of us. We all have our hearts broken during a lifetime to a greater or lesser degree. Just recognising a broken heart is where healing begins. Then you give yourself a space for the wounds and suffering of the past to be healed.

Some people are not consciously aware of having a broken heart because it happened when they were very small. Hearts – and spirits – can be broken during childhood by the actual loss of a parent through death or separation, or through the experience of loss when a parent or carer is absent, neglectful, abusive or conditional in their love. When our true and unique being is not reflected back to us in childhood, it can create a deep insecurity about our identity and self-worth. In adult life, these wounds can make themselves felt in behaviour such as compulsively searching to fill the unnamed aching void or addictions to work, substances, sex or love. This can put us at risk of heart disease.

Recognising a Broken Heart

If you find yourself responding to the image of the broken heart, try to get a sense of how or when you felt your heart got broken. Allow your heart to lead the way. You might find your-self remembering a difficult time of loss earlier in your life. You might see the image of a small child – yourself. Stay with the image or the memory and get a sense of what happened to your feeling heart.

♦ Did your heart go into the deep freeze?

♦ Did you decide never to trust anything to do with the heart ever again?

♦ Did you cut off from feeling, from vulnerability, and harden down?

♦ Did you go numb?

♦ Did you decide that one day you would get even?

♦ Did you push yourself into independence and action, vowing never to need anything or anyone ever again?

♦ Did you and your life go 'on hold', almost not daring to breathe or to live?

♦ Did you close off and fight any fragment of warmth or attachment?

♦ Did you begin a relationship with your heart, one that has led to a greater openness to life and other people?

This will give you a clue as to the nature of your 'coping strategies' for emotional pain. Spend some time now in considering how these coping strategies have served you. Are they still useful? If you feel they are, leave well alone. If not, it may be that they may have helped you survive a painful time in the past but may now be shutting you out of a vital connection to life. They may be adding to your physical and emotional stress.

Dying of a Broken Heart

Dying of a broken heart may be popular in verse, song and drama, but statistics show that this can be a physical reality. When we say someone 'died of a broken heart' we tend to refer to a person who never recovered from a life event that knocked the stuffing out of them. That life event is often associated with love in some way and with the connection and hope that love brings. This may be borne out in the 'little deaths' inside us whenever we are unable to find the connection with our true sense of ourselves or by the high incidence of physical deaths of bereaved spouses, especially those who have been married for a long time, in the first six months after their loss.

Closeness and intimacy help our well-being. People who are in relationships tend to have less heart disease than those who are alone or isolated, without support. The bond of love may include anger and arguments, but these are also communication about being alive. Being able to relate to others intimately may well be one of the best supports to protect us from heart disease and is vital for the process of recovery after a heart-related incident.

Grieving

No one ever told me that grief was like fear. I am not afraid, and yet I keep swallowing.

C. S. LEWIS, *A Grief Observed*

When someone we love dies or is lost to us in some other way we have to learn to live as a separate person. Grieving and mourning are important processes that everyone needs to engage with as a part of life. Grieving involves the heart all the time. The heart feels sore, heavy, wounded. 'There's a stone there now,' said one woman. Sometimes it's as if there's a hole where the heart was, or the heart feels pierced, stabbed, full of grit. And this is an actual physical feeling.

We may also carry the wounds of earlier bereavements that have not been recognised or mourned. This may be because they occurred when we were very small, because the deaths were so very hard to accept and so were buried, or the circumstances did not allow us to grieve. Our unresolved bereavement may be to do with an actual person who has died in the past, or with the death of an ideal, idea or way of life.

If you recognise unresolved bereavement, make a note of how this is being carried in your feeling heart – as coldness, anger, emptiness, and so on – and look up the exercises for this response (*see pages 25–7*).

There are bereavements and losses that seem cruel, 'heartless'. But love and losing go together, they are two sides of the same experience. The depth of our grief can be in relation to the depth of our love and ultimately this is what helps to heal the heart once again.

Grief is not linear but spiral. It's as if we venture towards the same place over and over and in different ways. The process is helped by having a language to describe our experience.

● EXPLORING THE BROKEN HEART

● What has broken your heart?

● What did you do then, or would you do now, with a broken heart?

● Who/what might help you heal or mend your broken heart?

● What could you draw upon that would be balm for your broken heart? What could you draw on from friendship, from your belief system, literature, nature, spiritual nourishment or your own inner resources?

● Make a note in your notebook of your responses to this exercise and take action to put nourishment into practice. Make a resolve to look after your broken heart more effectively.

JANET

Janet felt her heart was broken when her fiancé Tony died in a sailing accident two days before their wedding. They had known each other since childhood. Now in her late twenties, Janet found the loss unfair, even cruel. She had asked Tony not to go sailing that day as he was with a group of reckless friends. He had been the only one to die because he had been the last one to grab the lifejackets in an act of heroism. Janet's pain was made worse because both of them had had a strong Christian faith and Janet felt that she ought to grin and bear it now that Tony was with God. But inside she felt angry at him for going against her wishes and at the friends who had survived. She struggled with her faith, became depressed, overweight and almost reclusive, pouring all her attention into looking after her elderly mother.

Janet's angina began two months after her mother died. She was by then 51. When I met her it was as if she had given up on life, on love or attachment. The pain in her heart, diagnosed as angina, brought her professional help and seemed a sort of 'permission' to bring everything to the surface. Also, now her duties to her elderly mother were completed, it was as if fate had released her to give time to herself.

In talking about her life Janet released some of the pressure of her bitterness, anger and envy of others, and her guilt for these feelings. She began to think about how she might begin to live now. The armour around her heart began to loosen. She found it frightening at first but began to dream vividly and become interested in these dreams and their language. She was helped by attending workshops, learned the process of inner dialogue, and began attending prayer and meditation meetings and reading widely on different approaches to spirituality. As the months went on, her angina lessened. She still needed to have her heart monitored, but the young woman who had frozen up in unexpressed grief 20 years earlier started stepping out.

The Emptiness of the Broken Heart

When our heart is broken we feel we have no energy for life, everything is too much and our lives are empty. We long for something to fill our emptiness. This need can take us into desperate areas, none of which satisfy us. Being driven, we tend to become exhausted, which only deepens our hunger.

When Your Heart is Empty

If you feel your heart is empty, ask yourself:

♦ How long has my heart been empty?

♦ How am I trying to fill it?

Can you sit with the emptiness and not try and fill it until you know what needs to come into your heart?

When Your Heart isn't in It

Many experiences of depression are linked to the heart going out of life. If you dread the day and hate waking up, how can you deal with this differently?

♦ Try beginning the day by simply acknowledging what you feel – depression, gloominess, sadness, even dread. Tell yourself that you will continue with your day and plan to visit what you feel every hour. Then continue your day – going to work, cleaning the house, taking the dog out – trying to limit how much energy you give to the emotions around feeling depressed. Every hour, sit down and just acknowledge what you feel, not fighting it, not telling it to go away.

♦ Throughout the day notice the number of times you think in a depressed or avoidant way such as 'I'll never be able to...' or 'I won't do that now because I'm bound to fail...' Make a note of these times and count them up at the end of the day. It may be that habitual negative thinking is influencing your depressed feeling. You can revise this by subjecting your unhelpful thoughts to scrutiny such as 'Is it true I will fail just because I have in the past?'

♦ Experiment with staying 'fresh' in your attitude by practising just being in the present moment and see if this brings you some more space.

♦ If you recognise that you are depressed, have you told anyone about how you feel? Have you consulted anyone who might be able to help you with these feelings? (*See Resources, page 251.*)

♦ Look at all the areas of your life. If there are only certain areas that you don't have the heart for, is it time to rethink them?

A Broken Heart Turned Cold Heart

♦ Do you feel cold towards others?

♦ Do you feel that all your relationships turn to ice?

♦ Do others tell you that you give them the cold shoulder, that you are cold towards them? Now that you are stopping to consider this metaphor of the cold heart, what feelings might be influencing this coldness? Under the layer of ice is there hurt, fear or pride? Think about this reality if you resonate with the cold heart.

♦ What does your cold heart need? Does it need taking out of the deep freeze? How can you keep the warm blood flowing? What will help you with the thawing process?

♦ What would warm your cold heart?

A Heart Broken by Betrayal

♦ Did you once trust your heart to someone or something and have that trust betrayed?

♦ What was it you trusted that was betrayed?

♦ Have you trusted this aspect to anyone or to yourself since?

♦ If not, what still gets in the way?

♦ What would it take for you to take small steps towards trusting a person or experience?

♦ What do you need to let go of first?

♦ Can you forgive the past and let go of it in order to save your own heart now?

Wearing Your Heart on Your Sleeve

This expression originates from the troubadour tradition where a cloth heart bearing the image of a man's beloved was pinned on to his sleeve. It showed a woman that she was 'spoken for' and that the man was proud to declare his love. In today's more reserved culture we warn against 'wearing our hearts on our sleeves', as if the vulnerability this creates is to be avoided. However, it is a wonderful experience to meet people who do indeed wear their heart on their sleeve. Children do so most of the time and we are never in doubt as to their enthusiasms.

Do you wear your heart on your sleeve? If so, does it give you a sense of freedom and pleasure? Do you feel it is good for your heart – if so, keep open! Stay pleased to show your feelings, passions, excitement. Or are you wearing your heart on your sleeve in the hope of someone taking care of you? Do you feel vulnerable and needy all the time? Has this made you want to please others and do what they want in order that they will like or love you?

Often when we feel needy and unsure of our own worth, we try and mould ourselves on other people, particularly those in authority. Unfortunately the results of this are that we tend to get taken for granted, even used and abused, which leaves us even more vulnerable and likely to shut down.

So try to be aware of every time you say 'yes' when you mean 'no', or when you do something because someone else wants it and you hope it will lead to good things. Then begin to refuse when appropriate and give yourself the space for something else, something *you* choose. In this way you can remain open but not be exploited.

When the Broken Heart Becomes the Angry Heart

My tongue will speak the anger of my heart, or, my heart, concealing it, will break.

WILLIAM SHAKESPEARE, *The Taming of the Shrew*

Studies show that anger kills. This is anger, rage and hostility that finds no understanding and care within us and no place of expression. It can fill our heartspace with toxicity and hardens down the heart by driving up heart rate, blood pressure and cortisol and adrenaline, the blood chemicals associated with emotional stress.

Although it is usually given a bad press, because it is often used inappropriately, anger does not have to be lethal. It can be creative, focusing and cleansing. The appropriate expression of anger can literally get things off our chests. In his book *Anger: Wisdom for Cooling the Flames,* Thich Nhat Hanh gives exercises for being with our anger. We have drawn on his work on page 30.

Anger often gets buried when we do not realise we are angry or are not in a position to express it. Situations such as physical and emotional pain, discrimination, helplessness, powerlessness, being under the arbitrary control of others, humiliation, miscarriage of justice, being bypassed for promotion, or events beyond our control can lead to repressed anger.

Signs of Buried Anger

♦ Feeling tense, especially in the jaw, shoulders, chest; gritted teeth.

♦ Holding your breath.

♦ Withdrawing, freezing, going numb.

♦ Laughing, giggling, making a joke instead of saying what you really want to say.

♦ Turning the other cheek while feeling superior.

♦ Self-blaming – 'It must be my fault'.

♦ Self-denigrating – 'Never mind, I don't mind, I don't matter'.

♦ Smiling and placating, being extra nice for fear of losing favour.

♦ Going as far away as possible from a situation or person.

Acknowledging Your Anger

Have you ever acknowledged that you are angry?

♦ What are your associations with anger – from the past and the present?

♦ Do you recognise the times when you turn anger against yourself, in self-punishing schedules, self-negation?

♦ Are there times when you have angry outbursts?

♦ Do you try and 'control' anger anywhere, from anybody? If so, is this because you fear anger, at receiving it from others, at being angry yourself?

Once you recognise your own anger there are ways of accepting it. A safe way of expressing anger is first to acknowledge that you feel it. Then, if your anger has been fuelled because you never got the chance to voice it, you might like to express it by speaking of it out loud to yourself or a trusted friend or writing down your feelings. You can also write angry letters to those who have made you angry. Then you can destroy the letters in a ritual burning, thus letting go of all the anger. No one needs to be damaged by our understanding of our anger. It is ours – other people and the world simply offer hooks to draw it out of us.

> It is important to own the anger we feel, then not to feed anger by either focusing on it and fanning its flames or burying it in repressed rage.

● **MINDFULNESS OF ANGER**

This exercise helps you to simply stay with your feeling of anger and not get drawn into the emotions surrounding it.

* Allow the feeling of anger in your body – its potency, its deep feeling.

* Breathe in anger.

* Breathe out anger.

* Say to yourself:

'Hello my old friend. I know you are there.'
'I know that I am angry' or 'I have been angry.'
'I do not hide it or repress it. I know I am/have been angry.'
'I do not act out of anger.'
'I recognise anger's potency and let it inform my clarity of mind.'

The Open, Joyous, Compassionate Heart

In the wind something is fresh.
Spores from the arms of trees
bring life into the forest.
Ploughed fields are crisp
with the hard beauty of night frost.
Snowdrops pale green shoot is fearless.
Black auk can begin
winging its way to far off places.
Life begins again
allowing hope to turn the lens.
The green meadow glows.

ELIZABETH McCORMICK, 1996

Have you had experiences that made your heart sing? The heart may be broken but it is also a vehicle for positive, life-giving experiences and we are always free to choose our attitude. We may choose to see our broken heart as the end, drawing a line under it out of fear. Or we may choose to allow the suffering of our broken heart to invite us into a deeper relationship with ourselves.

Suffering can feel meaningless unless we choose to give it

the potential for meaning. When we say, in our hurt and pain, 'Why this, why me?', we take the first step towards a completely different relationship with suffering. Then we may find that other people have taken similar steps, that there is a well-trodden path before us that we never knew existed.

MARGARET

Margaret suffered an intense period of heartache after her baby granddaughter died. She had an inherited congenital malfunction that made it impossible for her heart and lungs to grow. Although Margaret had supported her son and his family throughout this experience, immediately afterwards they cut her off. Margaret said:

> I felt as if my heart was breaking, dying from utter grief, and I didn't know what to do. . . . The pain was enormous, relentless. Then I realised that my heart had pulled me into darkness to try and find the light inside the darkness.

The beginning of recovery came when Margaret was sent the poems of David White, *Poems of Self Compassion*, out of the blue by an acquaintance. Then she was listening to the radio one day and heard a story about a priest working with lepers, including a breathing practice which involves breathing out compassion. Finally she participated in the 'Order of Love' course organised by Barbara Stone.

> I took great heart from these things that had appeared to me spontaneously. I learned to work through the heart, giving myself and the family compassion. I would breathe into the pain. As I accepted it, it did not have to be there in the same quantity. I now feel strengthened. I'm better at self-compassion and compassion for others.

After four months Margaret's son suddenly telephoned her. She commented, 'It was as if the compassion and release had allowed his heart to move.'

Telling Stories

Much of our daily suffering is created by the stories we tell ourselves, stories based on the past and dominated by judgements and criticisms such as 'I'm no good', 'They are stupid' or 'It's not fair that...'

Stories also create the drives and tensions about the future such as 'When I've got that I will feel better' or 'When I've done that I'll be able to relax and be happy' or 'I must have this drink now because I can't bear the pain of not having it.' How often do we say, without thinking, 'I can't wait to...'? These types of story indicate that we are constantly postponing the possibility of having a full, relaxed and happy heart right now.

If we start noticing every time we pull ourselves back into the past or drag ourselves, and our promise of peace, into the future, we can begin living in the present moment – and put our heart into it. Start simply:

♦ If you are sipping a cup of tea, sip the tea and experience the tea.

♦ If you are washing up, feel your hands in the hot water, the satisfaction of cleaning the utensils that have served your food.

♦ If you are eating, eat slowly, after giving thanks for the food and the journey it has made to reach your plate.

Seeding a Spiritual Path

Many of the great sorrows in the world arise when the mind is disconnected from the heart. The heart allows for the stories and ideas, the fantasies and fears of the mind without believing in them, without having to follow them or having to fulfil them. When we touch beneath the busyness of thought, we discover a sweet, healing silence, an inherent peacefulness in each of us, a goodness of heart, strength and wholeness that is our birthright.

JACK KORNFIELD, *A Path with Heart*

Living in the present moment and reconnecting to your heart can bring a spaciousness in which you can find the seeds of spiritual life. These seeds are always there; all we have to do is to water them. As mentioned earlier, by 'spiritual life' we mean the simplicity of those experiences we may invite when we are free of attachment to world objects. For example, when we are walking by the ocean we have a completely different experience with each movement of each wave, each colour, each stone on the beach. The universe invites us into its beauty and magnificence that transcends the ordinary everyday.

Equally, once we have let go of attachment and the projections other people carry for us, and what we expect them to provide for us, we find a presence, a sense of communion so sweet it is like an exchange of precious nectar.

We may also have spontaneous experiences of spiritual awakening through what Abraham Maslow, one of the founding fathers of Transpersonal Psychology, called a 'peak experience'. This may be through a powerful, even overwhelming sense of 'otherness', an 'at-one-ness' with the world and all beings. It may be an experience of deep and utter darkness pierced by a great light. It may be an extraordinary dream or 'other life' experience. It may be through a near-death experience (*see also page 204–5*). These occurrences are not for 'striving after', but tend to emerge spontaneously, as a 'call', or when we have made the space for them, free from the clutter of emotional preoccupation and thought.

The Heart of Courage

In every spiritual tradition the heart is the most central, usually sacred and revered motif, and refers to the essence of divine nature of all beings. This heart is always with us whether we see it or not. It is always there for us to connect to, be nourished by, whatever we do or do not do. This heart is completely unconditional. In turn, this heart can equally be nourished by our attitude to its potential. Often this sense of heart begins to be awakened when what has been buried begins to ripen – often, as we have seen, through an emotional trauma of some kind.

It takes courage to move beyond the 'armoured heart' we may have developed in order to survive. This is the courage to remain open to something that feels emotionally painful when our tendency is to shut down on to emotion, to blank it out, take a pill, have a drink, go out and drive very fast. Courage begins the awakening process. The word 'courage' derives from the Latin for 'heart'. The heart was thought to be the seat of bravery, and also the seat of love. So the language itself offers us the image of courage and love coming together in the heart.

The courage to be loving towards yourself or other people means being open, and therefore defenceless, unarmoured, vulnerable. Keeping the heart open means that we take some risks with the unknown. This softens the heart so that we are more accepting of what is around us, more able to let go of our attachment to the material world, which can never fulfil the heart we long for.

Awakening the Compassionate Heart

What helps us to begin to allow and enjoy the healing silence within us is an attitude of loving kindness. In Buddhism it is called the practice of maitri. We need this loving kindness to create the fertile soul in which our individual spiritual life can grow.

> Every day, wherever you are, practise saying: 'May I be filled with loving kindness.'

We may use feeling as the gate that opens us up to a compassionate heart. This is not easy to do, but it is important to keep the idea of a heart filled with compassion as a potential light to guide us by, rather than something we have to strain to achieve. True compassion wants nothing for itself. It is not goal-orientated. It has no outcome other than well-being, peace of mind and happiness for everyone. When we look with true compassion at someone who is behaving badly and our heart opens to them, we send them loving kindness. The energy this encourages can be healing in itself, both to the giver and the receiver, where both are equal and sublime.

Discrimination and wisdom begin in the heart, with intimacy and honesty with yourself. If we follow a path with heart, we are following our true heart, not being led by the nose by lust, greed, a need for gratification, power or approval. Not only may we feel more in charge of our life and physical health, and more present in the moment, but we may well be open to giving and receiving compassion and love for all sentient beings. This offers a spiritual nourishment which is beyond price.

Chapter 2

UNDERSTANDING
THE ROLE OF STRESS

It is a poor heart that never rejoices.
NINETEENTH-CENTURY SAGE

W E BECOME STRESSED through our emotional reaction to life events, bringing the physical and feeling heart into intimate relationship with each other. There has been considerable research which shows that when our strategies for coping with the stresses of life become inadequate, the resulting excessive hormonal reactivity has a harmful effect on the heart and circulation. High blood pressure, coronary artery disease (angina and heart attacks), heart rhythm disturbances and even sudden cardiac death can all be the result of long-term inability to cope with stress.

Obviously there are other factors which predispose individuals to getting heart disease (called 'risk factors' by the medical profession). These are discussed in detail in Part 2. It is the combination of all these factors that have an effect upon the heart. Because many of our emotional reactions are learned, however, they can be revised. Our physical heart then does not have to take the strain of our emotions.

What is Stress?

Stress is a word that often produces fear and confusion. To feel stressed is to feel tense, out of control, trapped and, often, angry. Literally, stress means a stimulus or response. Each individual will have their own set of both biological and learned responses to experience. Riding a bicycle for one person may be associated with the open country road, good air, freedom and childhood picnics; for another it may mean terror, anxiety, struggle, exhaustion, pollution, busy main roads and the possibility of an imminent accident. Knowing how you become stressed and how you can manage stressful situations will make you feel more in control and will help your heart.

All of us need some stress – such as the early morning alarm clock – to get going. Healthy stress can be a positive motivation to continue with a project and see it through. So stress in itself is not a bad thing, since it can be the stimulus to achieve certain of our objectives.

Stress becomes a problem when the stressor is continuous, when we have no control over it or when our coping mechanisms become exhausted. Under such circumstances the strain exerted on the heart and circulation becomes harmful.

Coping Mechanisms

Coping mechanisms are the systems we use to deal with the various stressors in our lives. Some people have better coping mechanisms than others and all of us will respond to different stressors in different ways. Some people feel confident in their ability to deal with daily conflict, for example, and are strengthened by a row, while others may feel nervous, tentative, take conflict personally and feel criticised or even flattened by a disagreement.

Our own ability to cope can vary and while at certain times we can easily deal with stressors, on other occasions they may give us considerable difficulties. Everything we have to deal with in life takes more energy when we are recovering from an accident or illness, when we have lost a loved one or had a major change.

Some things are always stressful by their very nature – being under threat of redundancy, for example. When we are single and have skills we can offer elsewhere we will respond differently from when we have a family to feed, are getting older or finding our skills being replaced by technology. Similarly, a house move is always stressful because it involves physical, emotional and mental activity around change, but for one person this may be a long-awaited joy, for another a painful separation from the familiar.

If our coping mechanisms start to fail, it is easy to understand how a vicious circle may develop.

1. Knowing demands are being made on you, you feel stressed and try and cope as usual but things don't work out. You have no alternative coping strategies, so your anxiety remains high, you start to fear failure and nothing you do seems to have any impact upon your situation.

2. You try harder, in the same way, your anxiety rising as you see things slipping through your fingers. You begin to sleep badly, feel less able to concentrate. You might become bad-tempered and preoccupied. You work longer hours but achieve less.

3. You try to make changes, sometimes drastically – quit your job and/or relationship, change your appearance or even elect for a cosmetic operation, hoping this will be the 'magic bullet' to make you feel better – thus introducing other stressors on top of your existing stress. You have to strive harder than ever, perhaps turning to alcohol or drugs to sustain you.

4. If these procedures do not help resolve your situation, you begin to get more attached to the treadmill of stress. Everything you do ends up with you feeling hopeless, helpless, frustrated, ill and trapped. You begin to feel desperate,

panicky, and push on even harder, cutting out all your usual hobbies or friends.

5. You are now exhausted, prey to depression and negative thinking but trapped into carrying on. It's as if what once worked for you in the past no longer has any impact and you have no new ideas about coping. You are blinkered, worn out and have no energy to learn anything new. You reach a crisis point. The slightest thing can tip you over the edge and into breakdown and heart attack or stroke.

We may carry on in this way, seriously compromising our physical health, for several years until something 'breaks'. Doctors now recognise that the year before many heart attacks often contains prolonged maladaptive responses to stress which have pushed the heart beyond endurance. There are now recognised causal links between prolonged exhaustion (one year or more) and heart attack.

It is difficult for doctors to appreciate this problem because many of the symptoms of exhaustion are fairly non-specific. Some may be able to see the growth of unhealthy tension and symptoms of strain in their patients and be alert to the potential dangers. High blood pressure is one measurable symptom that is recognised as a potential response to stress.

Fortunately, you can learn to recognise when your stress level is too high before you become so stressed that your physiological as well as psychological heath is compromised. You can learn to recognise when your coping strategies are not working and to find new ones. The first step is to make an appraisal of your own level of stress.

Evaluating Your Stress

● STRESS ASSESSMENT

Take some time, either first thing in the morning, just after you wake, or at the end of your working day. Set aside 30 minutes for yourself.

Sit quietly in a comfortable place, on your own with no distractions such as radio, television, dogs, children or neighbours. Turn off the telephone. You might want to have a small notebook by your side so that you can write things down as they come to you.

First, just notice your breathing. Let it quieten down.

You are now going to explore how your whole system feels.

1. Ask your body how it feels

As before, use symbolic language – ask for an image, colour or shape. For example, if you get the image of a beached whale you may need to spend time with that whale finding out about it and what it most needs from you. It might be rest, or to get back into its own element (water), or to get to a place where it is less exposed. Ponder on how you might respond to this information.

After you have responded to your body's needs you might want to go a bit further. What is it that created the beached whale in your life? Can you learn to recognise the situation again, before it has grabbed your body in its force? What would help you to do this? What body signals are a forewarning of the beached whale to come?

Spend time monitoring how your body feels at different times of the day and in different situations – when driving, travelling, being at work, with certain people, at home, during hobbies. Get to know what situations help to nurture a sense of relaxation and put you in tune with your body; and which situations seem to build up tension and stress in your body.

2. Ask your mind how it feels

How does your mind feel? Again, can you find an image that expresses your thoughts? Sometimes, for instance, at the end of the day, if we have been using a lot of structured, logical thinking processes, our mind is like a swarm of bees buzzing for attention. If we allowed the swarm to take over, we would be stung. Diversion is badly needed. It may be cooking, a radio programme, a short walk, whatever supports the intent to switch off. (Becoming obsessional about exercise is not helpful here as it merely continues the process of overthinking and it is important not to exercise when you are fatigued, for this only demands more from the blood supply.) An obsessive mind that feeds on itself is not healthy. Here the most important action is to stop and rest.

3. Ask your heart how it feels

Are you carrying tension within your heartspace? If your heart feels heavy at the end of your day, what is in that heaviness? By exploring the nature of the image, can you reach a feeling? Once you have reached the feeling, can you spend time with it? Drawing, painting, writing about it or just sitting with it will help you to be in touch with the true nature of what you are feeling.

If your heartspace feels empty, what does the emptiness long for? Is your heart signalling that you need to be connected to something that raises your spirit, connects your soul to a source of nourishment? What might that be? Allow yourself to follow these ideas a little. Some people are nourished by soulful poetry or music that reaches into an empty heartspace in a warming and moving way.

● INNER AND OUTER DEMANDS

After you have taken 20 minutes to explore how you feel, what kind of overall picture do you have? You may feel tearful, depressed and angry that you are burdened and unsure what to do now, or you may feel happy that your life is supporting you. Whatever your outcome, you now need to look at the demands in your daily life and discover which are most stressful. Then you will be in a better position to see if you can do anything about them.

There are two kinds of demand that can subtly push us all into feeling stressed: the demands from outside – from others, our work and our environment – and the demands that come from inside us – from our attitude and our beliefs about ourselves.

Take another 10 minutes and draw a circle on a piece of paper. Put another circle in the middle to represent your potentially free, beautiful self – a self like no other. Around this, in segments, write down all the different aspects of your life – the roles you play, the demands on your energy from family, friends, work, interests, hobbies, home, garden, everything you can think of.

Now make plus or minus marks in each section to rate whether this area of your life gives you energy or takes it away (*see below*).

MAP OF EFFORT AND ENERGY BANK

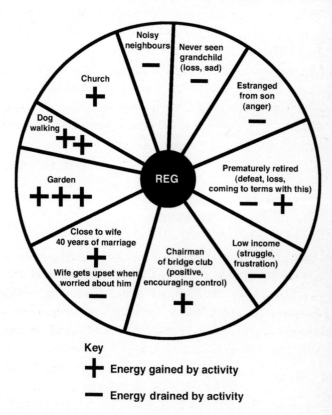

Key

+ Energy gained by activity

– Energy drained by activity

When you have your own map, pick out the area that is most demanding right now. Don't try and cover everything. And within this one area pick an aspect that you can begin to think about.

REG

Reg had a heart attack at 58, just after early retirement. He had been looking forward to retirement but the actuality was more difficult. Without realising it, he had become depressed and somewhat isolated.

Reg's energy map helped him to realise that being chairman of his bridge club and attending church both gave him energy. Using the energy gained from these two areas, he was able to go on to address one of the more painful areas of his life – his estrangement from his son. Reg and his wife spent some time discussing Reg's desire to re-establish contact with his son and this proved to be an opening for the family, for the two of them asked their son to come and visit with his new baby. It was the beginning of Reg feeling more in charge of his life and his levels of stress and, most important of all, being aware that he could evoke change.

One of the curious things about stressed people is that often they do not realise how stressed they are. They think it normal that they have to keep buying antacid tablets for indigestion, or something to help them sleep, to have a two-week headache or drown every evening in alcohol. There is an anecdotal story of one of Freud's early patients who, when asked to describe what he did on waking in the mornings, replied, 'Well, doc, the same as everyone else – I get out of bed, throw up into the basin, have a wash, get dressed and go to work.'

SABRES

To evaluate the stress you may be carrying, and whether it is at a healthy or unhealthy level, take a look at the following questionnaire, which is based upon the acronym SABRES. It was devised by Dr Peter Nixon when he was consultant cardiologist at Charing Cross Hospital, London. SABRES stands for Sleep, Arousal, Breathing, Rest and Effort, and Self-esteem.

Read through this section, making notes as you go. You might like to give yourself numbers out of 5, with 5 being the most stressful rating and 1 the least stressful.

Sleep

Sleep is our special place of restoration, the freest of all relaxation spas. It puts us in communication with our unconscious, so that the riches of our inner world may be revealed. Often, however, we do not consider our sleep, and asking about the quality of sleep is left to psychologists when assessing clinical depression. Let's look at how you sleep.

♦ Is your sleep natural, restful? Do you wake feeling rested and alert, ready for the day? (This would be a 1.)

♦ Do you wake early, around 3 a.m., and then toss fretfully about?

♦ On waking, do you feel exhausted, as if you'd not had any sleep?

♦ Do you lie awake until the early hours and then find yourself unable to wake up in the morning?

♦ How long is it since you noticed your dreams? Dreams can give you useful information about your inner life. Find someone you might talk to about your dreams so that you might understand them. The release of energy through dreams can be cathartic and healing. (*See also pages 231–2.*)

♦ Do you have disturbing dreams or nightmares? Do you know what they are trying to tell you?

♦ Do you have to take sleeping pills, tranquillisers, cough medicine or calming herbal remedies?

♦ How do you feel about sleep? Are you afraid to go to sleep? Are you afraid that you won't sleep?

♦ Ponder on when was the last time you slept naturally and well and woke feeling refreshed. What was going on during that period? Who was around? What were you doing? How were you feeling?

♦ Ponder now upon the themes of your life that could be affecting your sleep. Have you got into the habit of eating late, staying up late, avoiding going to bed and not sleeping? Can you work out what you might be avoiding?

Accepting Wakefulness

Sometimes, during major changes, and especially during and after a serious illness or an event such as a heart attack, our sleep is affected. It is possible that this is a sort of protection for our sense of self. When something major is occurring we do not want to be asleep; we need to be awake. Conversely, our bodies and minds also desperately need the rest sleep can bring.

Just knowing that we are moving through an important and transitional period of time can help us accept a difficult sleep pattern. In order to accept wakefulness, rather than fight it, you need to make use of it.

So, choose one of the following options, or try each out on different nights.

1. Get up and make tea, read, walk around and be active for a set time (say, half an hour to an hour) rather than lie and ruminate and possibly exaggerate your emotional tensions.

2. Lie very still and concentrate upon your breathing, the in and out rhythm, like the rise and fall of a gentle ocean tide. Each time you find a thought dominating the space in your mind, just release it, let it go and return to the breath. Sometimes we are helped to continue focusing on the breath by bringing in a 'breath poem' or an image. A 'breath poem' is similar to 'I have arrived, I am home', something very short that helps to bring us back to our breath. The use of an image is to help our concentration and to still

the chattering mind. You might like to choose an image that you find particularly peaceful, such as a rose, a lotus or an evergreen tree, and concentrate upon its colour, shape and fragrance.

If you feel that your sleep is compromised, it is advisable to seek professional help. Talk to your doctor about sleeping or tranquillising medication or natural herbal remedies to help you with sleep. It's important not to let sleep disturbances become an enemy.

Arousal

Arousal is another word for stress. When we have been living in a state of stress for a long time many of our body systems become compromised. Arousal describes the state of the body organs and systems that are under stress.

Do you suffer from any of the following? Give yourself 5 for 'often', 3 for 'sometimes', 1 for 'occasionally' and 0 for 'never'.

♦ Acid stomach.

♦ Constant swallowing, dry mouth.

♦ Stiff neck and jaw.

♦ Back pain.

♦ Poor diet – can't be bothered to buy healthy food.

♦ Either eating compulsively or not eating regularly.

♦ Headache.

♦ Constipation.

♦ PMS, period pain and irregularity.

♦ Muscular or joint pain.

♦ Avoidance of exercise because you 'can't be bothered'.

♦ A permanent fearful, anxious state.

♦ A short fuse.

♦ Ideas of escape, a wonderful future without any responsibility.

♦ The postponing of happiness.

♦ Dreams of aeroplane crashes, lifts falling, running to catch a moving train.

If your score is over 45 Your body and organs are highly aroused. You need to start immediately to work on lowering your levels of stress. Take as much time as you can and just *stop*. Do some simple relaxation and breathing exercises *(see page 211)*. Make sure that you get a night of proper sleep every day of the week. Make an energy map for yourself *(see page 43)* to assess which area of your life is the most problematic. Find someone to talk to about your personal stress. Consult your medical practitioner, giving specific details about your condition as you have now observed it.

   If your score is between 25 and 45 You have high to moderate stress and could benefit from all the procedures outlined above. Try a mild exercise programme if you are fit enough to walk one mile. Go for the walk however you feel emotionally. You may find that as you attend to relaxation and breathing your other symptoms improve. If you feel concerned, consult your medical practitioner for more advice about your personal stress levels.

   If your score is between 10 and 25 You are mildly stressed and need to pick one area that you can improve on.

   If your score is under 5 You are relaxed – congratulations!

Hurry Sickness

When someone is aroused by stress they tend to have a swollen, 'eyes on stalks' look about them and to walk like a heron, with their head and neck stretched out in advance. Impatience and irritability at small things may quickly escalate into rage followed by weeping. Last of all, and biggest by far because it seems endemic, is 'hurry sickness'. This is a state of always being on the run.

Perhaps you find yourself with piles of paper that are never read. The piles grow, adding to your frustration, panic and sense of work building rather than ending. You keep saying 'I'll catch up with that this evening/in bed/on the loo...', but you never do. You may take things on but cannot finish them because you start the next thing first. You may have an illusion of lots happening in your life but that you are losing control and cannot stop. It is as if you are unconsciously waiting for something to stop you – something external like an accident or event happening to another person that involves you, or something internal such as a heart attack, breakdown or illness that finally brings you to a halt.

If this sounds like you, Chapter 16 explains how to deal with stressors and avoid being brought suddenly to a halt.

Breathing

What is your pattern of breathing like? Spend tomorrow just noticing your breathing at different times, during meals, when you are talking, using the telephone, walking, sitting on a train or on the bus. Notice what changes your breathing. Is it activity or is it emotion? If it is emotion, which emotion is it? What are your associations with that emotion and what does it make you feel? (*See also pages 10–11.*)

When you are stressed, you can get used to holding your breath in the same way as you are holding on to your life, trying to stay in control when you feel that control slipping or when you are afraid. Then you have to gulp for air or give long sighs or even hyperventilate. It's as if you cannot give yourself time for basic breathing.

One of the small, most useful techniques for remaining free of stress is diaphragmatic breathing. It is also useful for managing fear in cases of angina and heart failure, where the fear produces the adrenaline, which makes us breathe faster, which makes us afraid, and so the unhealthy cycle is perpetuated.

If you can notice your breathing regularly you will stay in balance with your body, mind, emotions and spirit. 'Going back to the breath' at demanding times was a life-saving habit for my husband John (McCormick) during his 22 years of living with heart disease. Even in intensive care, after pneumonia and for the short time he was off a ventilator, he practised the abdominal breathing that had supported him all his life since his heart attack.

● GOING BACK TO THE BREATH

● Wherever you are, stop whatever you are doing and place your hands on your lap if sitting or gently on your abdomen if lying or standing.

● Close your eyes and focus your attention on the breath and where you imagine the breath to enter the body. It might be just below the nostrils, the throat or the abdomen.

● As you breathe in, note the passage of air entering and filling your lungs and body cavities.

● Then, on the out-breath, follow the breath down as it leaves the body and your chest deflates. As far as possible allow this out-breath to be the longer breath and let there be a space at the end of it before allowing the breath to enter the lungs and body once more.

● Repeat this for five minutes.

During this process you should not feel breathless or struggle for air. If you do, concentrate upon relaxing your chest and shoulder muscles, keeping your focus of attention on the breath itself as it gently moves in through the nostrils or mouth and begins its passage through your entire body.

● USING A BELL

Try a test for yourself. Buy a series of automatic timers and set them to go off throughout the day. Whenever you hear the bell (and the telephone can be included), stop whatever you are doing and go back to the breath. Breathe three times, slowly – in then out. Each time the bell calls you, stop and return to this still point, just for three breaths.

Thich Nhat Hanh teaches that this simple practice of going back to the breath throughout the day helps us to develop mindfulness and then relaxation and peacefulness, whatever is going on around us. His own work began and grew throughout the war crisis of Vietnam.

See if this simple exercise has an impact upon your day and how you feel. If you are interested in knowing more about the practice of mindfulness, *see page 213.*

Rest and Effort

Rest means those times when whatever we are doing restores or gives us energy. Sometimes our work gives us energy, particularly when it is going well and we have accomplished something. Going for a walk, planning a surprise and being understood by someone are all energy-givers and therefore restful and restorative for our system as a whole. Resting does not have to be limited to taking a nap in the afternoon, lying or sitting down, relaxation or listening to music.

Effort means everything that we do – talking, taking a bath, making a cup of coffee, travelling to work, or making decisions, however small. Each of us needs to evaluate for ourself the effort required to do different things in our daily routine. What may be easy for one person might be difficult for another. Also, during difficult times, for example after illness or shock and during changes in our life, our usual routine takes more energy than when we are well and things are going along at their usual pace.

● ENERGY BALANCE

● Take a notebook and on one page make two columns.

● In the left-hand column write all the activities that required effort yesterday. Use a score from 1 to 5 to indicate the level of effort required, using 5 for a high effort requirement.

● In the right-hand column write down activities that gave you energy – talking to a kind friend, going swimming, taking a walk, hearing a good radio programme, writing a letter you've been meaning to write for ages. Score the level of energy you gained from each activity.

● When you add up the figures, you will see whether there is an energy deficit, a plus or a balance for the day.

● Continue this process for a week so that you can see the checks and balances of your life and its demands.

This pattern will show you the activities in your life that are draining your energy and need to be revised. It will also help you to plan future activities so that you do not crowd too many things into one day and that effort is followed by rest.

During times of low energy we need to give ourselves permission to rate the energy in our balance as being low. I (Elizabeth) often ask patients how much is there in the energy bank. They will take a few moments to consult their body and feelings and then may reply that there is 35 per cent. Then we might discuss priorities for that 35 per cent so that the body and feelings do not become even more compromised. It is often a relief to feel that you do not have to go on endlessly pushing yourself, having recognised that the balance of energy is simply not there.

Establishing a good balance of rest and effort supports a healthy system. It means that we can work very hard and then take an equal time to restore our balance.

♦ Is your hard day's work followed by a decent evening of relaxation and a good night's sleep?

♦ Do you regularly take time out for yourself?

♦ If you don't, how can you plan some rest times and restore your energy bank?

Self-esteem

Lack of self-esteem is the most frequent difficulty in patients who consult a counsellor or therapist. It may be something we are not actually aware of because it is hidden in attitudes we take for granted. We may have become accustomed to thinking that we don't really matter or are not worth much and that there's not much point in looking after ourselves. Some people also think that it's selfish to think about yourself. Many of us make harsh judgements about ourselves all of the time, thus restricting our choices of being in the world and adding to our stress.

Developing self-esteem means learning to become self-aware enough so that we know how to look after ourselves and plan a life where we really understand our own nature and how to live healthily with our hearts.

Placation

♦ Do you feel you have to please other people and do what they want?

♦ Do you feel taken advantage of by others, which makes you depressed and angry?

♦ Are you uncertain about yourself and your rights?

This pattern of pleasing others is called 'the placation trap' in psychotherapy. It is a trap because it doesn't lead anywhere. It usually develops in our early life where we have to agree to others' demands regardless of what we feel in order to survive.

Fortunately, with age and revision these learned survival habits can be changed, and our self-esteem raised.

● ESCAPING THE PLACATION TRAP

If you feel you are in the placation trap, spend a week monitoring the times when you say 'yes' when inside you are saying 'no'. Then start asking yourself what would happen if you started to say 'no'. You may fear that you will be rejected if you don't say 'yes', and yet as long as you are not saying what you really feel, the acceptance you seek is conditional and others have power over whether you feel OK or not. Try some small challenges to the old pattern such as saying 'I'm not sure about this, I need some time to think about it' and see what happens, both in yourself and in the other person.

Worthlessness

Often when we feel worthless we think there's no point in doing anything. We believe that even if we do try something we will do it badly. Often thinking in this depressed way leads to us feeling depressed. This can lead to us avoiding contact with others and becoming isolated and then our low self-esteem has no chance of revision.

Sometimes we feel we cannot have what we want because if we do we will be punished; others will reject or abandon us; or everything we get is bound to go wrong or sour anyway. This makes us turn in on ourselves and give up trying – we are defeated before we even start. Some people even think that their heart problems are a sign that they are no good or are to be punished and it proves that they should never have expected anything else.

● CHANGING YOUR RESPONSE

Many of these patterns are learned early in our life and while they may have helped us to survive then, when they are no longer useful to us it is time to revise them.

If these patterns of thinking are very familiar to you, there are several things you can do:

* Record the nature of your thinking in your notebook.

* Discuss these patterns with a trusted professional, a nurse or doctor, or a friend.

* Decide to take time to find a psychological counsellor or therapist who will help you to revise the pattern of worthless thinking that has eroded your sense of self-esteem.

Your heart may be the 'awakener' to these problems with self-esteem. As it opens, you have 'permission' to receive care and to allow something good to come into your life.

In Buddhist philosophy, all of us already have everything that we need inside us, it's just that we don't see it. Listening to ourselves and becoming aware of the patterns that restrict us is where we begin to relieve ourselves of suffering. Accepting change is the next step; releasing love, joy and the capacity to feel connected is the third step.

All of us have periods when our self-esteem is challenged. What is important is your awareness of yourself as a whole person with positive and negative experiences and aspects. Both need to be included in your acceptance of yourself and in turning your attention to the needs of your heart.

Read Your Heartspace

It will help you to remain in touch with your level of stress if you learn to 'read' your heartspace on an everyday basis, because this is where many of your difficulties will first be located.

Very often it is the breath itself that guides us and shows us the way to both recognise and dissolve the hardest of emotional tangles that may be pressing on our heartspace. This process allows our preoccupations, worries and fears to be taken away from the chest and into practical solution in our life. Breathing in to the area of pain or difficulty and breathing out into the world once again and differently is one way of addressing this demand upon the heartspace. Knowing what is on your chest as well as 'getting it off your chest' is freeing for the heartspace physically and emotionally. (For breathing exercises, *see pages 49, 50 and 211*.)

Stressful Events

Obviously some events are more stressful than others and all of us experience times when our rating on the SABRES questionnaire above will be severely compromised. When we realise we are stressed, we need to evaluate where this response to stress is really coming from. This will be a mixture of the stressors and our attitude towards them.

According to the often quoted Holmes and Rahe stress scale inventory, the most stressful event is the death of a spouse. Other highly stressful events include divorce, taking on a mortgage, moving home, and any changes in circumstances, even Christmas. But in addition to all these external events we need to take our individual coping skills and attitudes into consideration. What might be stressful for one person, such as flying in an aeroplane, will be exciting for another. And change is both exciting and frightening.

Assessing Your Personal Stressful Events

Make a list of the five areas in your life that have been the most stressful during the last two years – for example, moving house or job, giving up work, children leaving home, change in diet or recreation, serious illness and death of close friends or relatives, worry over money and housing, or having to deal with complex new information, with the law, injustice, or sexual or racial harassment and discrimination.

♦ How did you cope? Did you battle on alone or find support, or was it a time full of chaos and confusion?

♦ What helped you through? (For example, listening to music or relaxation tapes or talking to friends.)

♦ What is left outstanding that you would like cleared up?

♦ Might you be able to bring that about now to relieve the burden of the event?

♦ If you met with these circumstances again, what would you do that was different?

JOHN
While travelling in Africa, John's angina increased. Instead of trying to ignore it or rushing to take glyceryl trinitrate (GTN) he first of all sat down immediately and breathed in a controlled, orderly fashion, which he had previously learned (*see pages 214–15*). He picked up the pre-signalling signs for angina each time it was about to occur again and stopped travelling before an attack came on. The pace of the rest of his journey was organised to suit his need for rest and effort so that angina was avoided.

Try rating your stress level as it was and how it is now by consulting the SABRES list above and evaluating your response to the past stressful times in this way.

In the section below we have tried to explain some of the mechanisms by which the stressors that you are experiencing may affect your heart. Later we have given some tools to ameliorate the effects.

The Chemistry of Stress

As social animals, we have a complex hierarchy and continuously compete for control and status. When power is used well, there is harmony and learning. When power is used corruptly, discriminately or arbitrarily, those serving under the system become stressed. Often this is seen in fear of losing position and income, anxiety over how to respond and frustration when the response has no recognition.

If you think there is a threat to your sense of environmental control, you struggle to re-establish and maintain better control. During this time, you will actively make an effort and you will experience a release of noradrenaline. As long as there is no fear, your adrenaline levels probably remain the same or even decline. At some point you may give up and become passive, perhaps exhausted by the effort, and this makes your cortisol levels rise. These hormones have a very important role in setting the stage for heart disease. And this powerful pattern, of struggling to gain control over circumstances followed by collapsing into giving up, is repeated over and over again during a lifetime.

Hyperventilation

The increase in the breathing rate that occurs as part of your response to your emotions can continue inappropriately and cause all kinds of dramatic physical sensation, including shortness of breath (difficulty getting enough air into the lungs, frequent sighing and gasping breaths), chest pains and palpitations, tingling in the hands and feet, tremors, giddiness, faintness and nausea.

Hyperventilation can be seen in its most acute form as part of phobic anxiety, for example the panic associated with claustrophobia. In such cases the dramatic overbreathing with short, shallow, fast breaths causes very unpleasant symptoms. The symptoms are due to a lowering of carbon dioxide (which is exhaled with each breath) and such acute attacks are best dealt with by breathing into a paper bag, which brings the level of carbon dioxide back towards normal.

Hyperventilation can also occur chronically. It may become the dominant pattern of breathing. Instead of slow, regular breaths with the *abdomen* rising and falling with each breath, only the top part of the chest is used. The breathing rate increases and the level of carbon dioxide falls. This causes many symptoms that can mimic or even exacerbate heart problems.

This type of breathing pattern appears to be learned, perhaps in response to panicky or stressful situations, or following abdominal operations or pregnancy. Sometimes we learn to 'puff out the chest' when in the army or when asked to 'sit up straight' or 'put our backs into something'. Sometimes a raised chest is a physical sign of our having to act 'big and brave' at times when we really did not feel like it, and the pattern in our body got stuck. These habitual body postures often promote upper chest breathing patterns, which lead to hyperventilation.

Treating this type of breathing pattern is very important, as is understanding the underlying causes.

● TREATING HYPERVENTILATION

- Place one hand, palm down, on the abdomen.

- Place the other hand, palm down, on the upper chest.

- When breathing in, try to make the hand on the abdomen move up and down while keeping the hand on the chest still.

It will be possible to slow the breathing down to about 12 breaths per minute.

It is important to practise breathing in this way at all times, particularly when under stress. In addition it is important to breathe this way when exercising – sometimes people become worried when starting exercise and hyperventilate as a result, which reduces their performance.

Hyperventilation can give rise to palpitations, chest pain and other heart symptoms even when there is no heart disease present. The chest pain is often sharp and may be under the left breast at about the fifth rib. It may even be tender here. Sometimes the joints of the ribs with the sternum may also be tender. Hyperventilation mimics heart disease so well that it has been found in 67 per cent of people with normal coronary arteriograms (X-ray examination of the coronary arteries).

Hyperventilation can also be the pattern of breathing when there *are* heart problems and may compound them. The lowered carbon dioxide levels constrict arteries and if there is already a narrowing in a coronary artery for example, it may make angina worse or bring it on earlier. In addition hyperventilation increases the heart rate and so again may make the angina worse. At least 55 per cent of patients seen in one cardiac rehabilitation programme were found to hyperventilate. Of these about one-third were found to hyperventilate with activity, half when discussing emotive topics and the remainder as a habit.

> Hyperventilation is a major problem and should be addressed. With training and practice habitual hyperventilation can be overcome.

Combatting Stress

There are several shorthand ways you can use to cope with stress and resist any illness that might result from a stressful lifestyle.

Hardiness

Hardiness develops from knowing yourself and your reactions to inner and outer demands and being able to commit yourself to keeping a still centre within and standing firm when life is testing. The still centre may be developed by using some of the self-help techniques outlined throughout this book – getting to know yourself and your responses, relaxing, practising breathing techniques, undertaking a healthy exercise programme and learning the practice of mindfulness (*see page 213*).

Eating a healthy diet (*see page 220*) and developing a supportive social network that includes friendship, laughter, fun, recreational hobbies and activities also contributes hugely to our well-being and capacity to maintain a still centre. Being involved in a community project or in the responsibility for others' care also creates healthy links.

You can incorporate these elements into your life and build a good resistance to harmful stress by following three 'C's: Commitment, Control and Challenge.

♦ **Commitment** Becoming actively involved in what is going on, rather than withdrawing, means you are supporting your self-esteem, sense of meaning and belonging, and are less prone to depression and defeat.

♦ **Control** The ultimate freedom is to choose your own attitude. No one can take this away from you. Taking a positive view and taking charge of what you can be in charge of is preferable to feeling passive and helpless. This does not mean a naïve or omnipotent expectation of being completely in charge of all events and outcomes. It means that through the exercise of imagination, knowledge, skill and choice you can direct your energy more effectively, whatever the outcome. In terms of coping, a sense of control leads to an action aimed at transforming events into something consistent with what you need. It appears to be responsible for the development of a broad and varied repertory of responses to stress.

♦ **Challenge** You should encourage yourself to believe that change rather than stability is normal in life and that the anticipation of change is an interesting incentive to growth rather than a threat to security. Challenge fosters openness and flexibility.

Mindfulness

We may extend our awareness of our breathing into a more extensive practice called mindfulness of breathing. The practice of mindfulness brings our concentration to the simple act of breathing, just concentrating on the nature of the in-breath and the out-breath. We may also become mindful of our everyday activities such as taking a shower, washing up, cleaning, working in the garden or at our jobs, eating, and so on. We simply focus our attention on the task we are doing – breathing in, I wash the dish, breathing out, I put the dish on the side – and try to avoid our mind scattering in different directions, into the past or future. The practice originates from the ancient tradition of Zen Buddhism and thus is a well-practised, well-researched way of bringing a sense of peace, stillness and well-being to our entire body, mind and emotions. The space and lightness created by mindfulness practice also have the potential to move your awareness into the spaces that offer spiritual nourishment.

Mindfulness or meditation practised regularly is a way of being very still. The stillness helps us to appreciate what our bodies and psyches are carrying. Regular practice keeps us in touch with our own personal space, a space free from distraction, purpose, agenda. It is like an island within ourselves, a pure space within which we may live and breathe, whether we are in the middle of a volcano or just struggling with the daily grind.

JULIAN
Julian began to have tight, painful feelings in his chest while walking on the beach after lunch at the pub. It was winter and cold. He was an experienced meditation practitioner

and knew how to relax around pain, just breathing in to it to take the panic out of it. The pain lasted about 20 minutes, but was alarming and Julian went to the doctor a couple of days later.

During a week of resting and taking things very slowly, Julian found that even the smallest stress would trigger pain in two particular places, just to the side of the chest. His doctor sent him straight into hospital. Julian recalled:

> They were in a quandary, because I didn't have a proper symptoms pattern with which they could identify. But rather than wait and see, they threw every potion and pill at me – beta blockers, GTN and pills to reduce cholesterol and aspirin to thin the blood. I got this tag of 'difficult patient' because I asked so many questions about the pills and whether there were alternatives. It took a lot of screwing up of my power to get out of the hospital.

Julian had not had a heart attack and did not have underlying heart disease. His problems were related to stress. He was helped by Chinese medicine and cranial osteopathy.

> I'd been going through a period of extraordinarily high stress. In the space of two years six friends had died, then on top of that we had the whole breakdown of my partner's family. Every time you turned your back there was another great big unsolvable drama and they went on and on. It was terrible. And what had precipitated this particular attack of chest pain was that the previous night I'd been out on a binge and drunk too much, which had affected the liver, and in Chinese medicine the liver is connected to the pericardium around the heart. A Chinese herbalist treated the liver and a cranial osteopath treated me as well. She put her hand on my foot and said, 'Something's happened to you. It feels as if

something's almost scared you to death.' Just being recognised in this way was healing.

For a period of time Julian's pains continued because he couldn't just switch off the stress as it was at such a high level. But he learned to calm down and take better care of himself.

PART TWO

Understanding the Physical Heart and Heart Problems

Chapter 3

THE PHYSICAL HEART

The mind has a thousand eyes
And the heart but one...
F. W. BOURDILLON, *Among the Flowers 'Light'*

THE BEATING HEART was once considered the most mysterious, sacred and untouchable aspect of a person. It was thought to be the house of the soul and the property of a god.

The heartbeat is still special. It is the first sign of life in the unborn child. We take someone's pulse to ensure they are still alive. In Chinese medicine the five pulses around the wrist area give information about the well-being of all the internal organs, of which the heart is sovereign.

The beating heart also has symbolic meanings – politicians may speak of the nation's heartbeat, for example. Every kind of music echoes different beats that can correspond with our current mood and emotional need – when we feel the pulse, we groove into the rhythm.

When the heartbeat, whether physical or symbolic, is manifest, life pulsates. When there is no heartbeat, life, in the form we know it on Earth, ceases.

The heart beats about 30 million times a year. There is no other piece of engineering that does this without rest.

The Heart and its Function

The Four Chambers of the Heart

The heart is situated just beneath your breastbone (sternum) with the apex pointing leftwards beneath your left nipple. It is a system of chambers linked by valves. There are collecting areas above each pump (ventricle) where blood is kept in readiness to fill the pump. These are called the left atrium and right atrium (atrium comes from the Latin meaning 'hall'). For efficiency, there are four 'no-return' valves in each pump. On

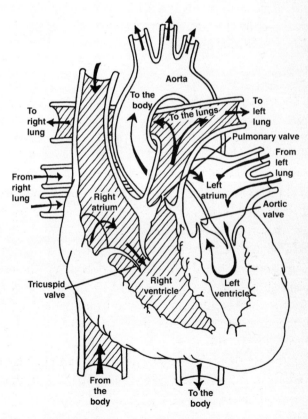

How the Heart Functions
The right side of the heart receives deoxygenated blood from the body through the pulmonary vein and sends it to the lungs. The left side receives oxygenated blood from the lungs and sends it to the body via the aorta.

the left side, the one between the left collecting chamber (left atrium) and the left pump (left ventricle) is called the mitral valve; the one between the left ventricle and the main artery to the body (aorta) is called the aortic valve. On the right side, the one between the right collecting chamber (right atrium) and the right pump (right ventricle) is called the tricuspid valve; the one between the right ventricle and the main artery to the lungs (the pulmonary artery) is called the pulmonary valve.

The Coronary Arteries

The heart itself also needs oxygenated blood and this comes through the coronary arteries, so called because they form a pattern like a coronet around the heart.

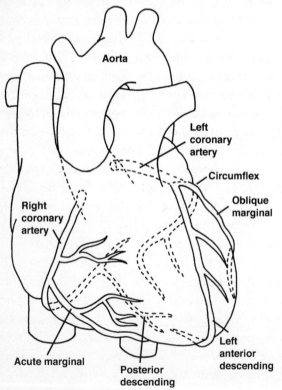

The Coronary Arteries
The positions of the coronary arteries around the heart.

The right coronary artery supplies the underside or inferior part of the heart. The left coronary artery has a big main trunk from which two major divisions occur. The front or anterior of the heart is supplied by the left anterior descending coronary artery; the other artery curls around to supply the areas in between the other arteries and is called the circumflex.

Because they are quite small, the coronary arteries are often affected by atherosclerosis, a disease process which thickens the walls of the arteries. A heart attack is caused when a coronary artery becomes blocked, hence the expression 'coronary' or 'coronary thrombosis' when this occurs.

Blood Pressure

Each time the pump (ventricle) pushes blood out it creates a surge of pressure to distribute the blood around your body to the different organs. The peak of this pressure is called systolic pressure. You can feel this surge of pressure in your own pulse. The ventricle works by contracting its specialised muscle (called the myocardium), and when it relaxes, new blood fills the ventricle. The baseline pressure in the system to which it falls back after the surge created by the contraction of the heart muscle is called diastolic pressure.

To visualise this process, imagine an ocean wave building up enough pressure to break into white water on to the beach. Then picture the return drag of water on the sand or stones as the wave cycle gets ready to repeat.

Doctors measure the pressure in the system using a blood pressure cuff (sphygmomanometer) which records the peak and trough against a column of mercury. Thus the pressure surge (systolic pressure) is recorded first and the baseline pressure (diastolic pressure) second. A typical reading might be 120 systolic and 80 diastolic and is conventionally referred to as 120 over 80 and written as 120/80. Your blood pressure varies from minute to minute depending on your levels of activity and the time of day.

The Cardiovascular System

Oxygen: the Essence of Life

Blood circulates in order to bring oxygen to the body. No part of the body could survive without this basic necessity. You probably know what it feels like if there is a lack of oxygen, for example in an overfilled or smoke-filled room, or if you climb to over 3,000 metres – you slow down, every movement requires a huge effort and you may also feel light-headed and nauseous.

Oxygen is carried in the bloodstream on red blood cells. Every part of your body is supplied with blood through an ever-diminishing network of arteries. When the blood reaches an organ, the arterial network subdivides still further into tiny channels called capillaries. Oxygen is then exchanged across the walls of the capillaries so that the organ may function properly with its fresh supply of oxygen. Once this is done, the

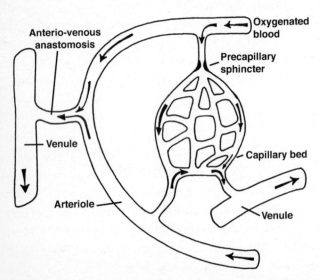

The Capillaries
The capillaries are the final pathway of fine vessels delivering oxygenated blood to every part of the body. The deoxygenated blood, containing carbon dioxide and other unwanted products, is then taken away from the capillaries via the venules, which are part of the venous return system to the heart and lungs.

blood flows away and is collected from the capillaries into the return system called veins, which get progressively bigger as they return to your heart and lungs. The blood takes away with it carbon dioxide and other unwanted products from the organ.

The Interaction between Heart and Lungs

The blood is pumped around your body by your heart, which moves 5,000 gallons of blood every day. There are two separate pumps in your heart, which work in tandem. The left pump (or ventricle) pushes oxygenated blood to the main artery in the body (aorta). The right pump (or ventricle) pushes blood with carbon dioxide in it to your lungs.

As you breathe in and out, your lungs allow the exchange of oxygen for carbon dioxide. The right ventricle sends blue blood (with carbon dioxide) to the lungs to allow this to take place. Then red blood (with oxygen) is sent to your left ventricle and on to your body.

In this way heart and lungs are vitally linked. In the resting state they are usually nicely balanced. To allow activity to take place, breathing and heart rate will both increase. Sometimes, however, one or other can get out of synch and this can cause problems.

Heart Rhythms: the Electrical System of the Heart

The heart needs an electrical stimulus to make it work. In fact the heart is very special in that any of its cells can generate an electrical impulse, albeit at different speeds. In order for this to be coordinated, however, there has to be a 'leader of the orchestra' that dictates the speed of the heart. This is called the sino-atrial (SA) node and is situated in the right atrium. The electrical impulse from this area spreads down to a substation called the atrioventricular node, which is found at the junction between the atrium (collecting area) and the ventricle (pump). From here the impulse is sent down two very fast pathways called the bundles of His which make the right ventricle and left ventricle contract.

The heart rate varies in each individual from minute to minute and at different times of the day, just like the blood pressure. At rest it can be between 50 and 70 beats per minute and with activity it can go up to 170 or more.

Sometimes one of the other areas of the heart decides to start a heartbeat a little earlier, after which there is a pause as the heart resets to the dominant rhythm. During the pause more blood fills the heart and so the next beat often feels more forceful (like a thud) and is called an ectopic. These beats do

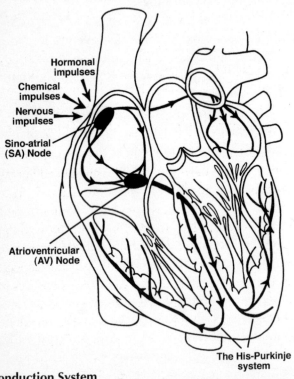

The Conduction System

The sino-atrial node initiates the heartbeat and sends an impulse to the atrioventricular node. Very rapid impulses are then sent down the His-Purkinje system to make the heart beat. Chemical, hormonal and nervous effects control the rate of the heartbeat.

not usually present problems, although they can feel quite uncomfortable. Sometimes taking a big breath or moving around can stop them. (*See page 106.*)

Effort and the Heart

The heart's main function is to provide for physical, emotional, mental and psychological effort. Your capacity for effort influences everything you do in your daily life. When you are slowed down by ill health, you become aware of how much effort it takes to make even small movements.

There is also the hidden effort of your autonomic nervous system, which operates your breathing, pumps blood around the heart, brain and body, and enables your liver, kidneys and digestive system to function.

The requirements of your body's organs for oxygen change frequently through the day in response to factors such as exercise, emotion or sleep. The circulation of blood to these organs has therefore to be able to respond to a number of circumstances and is controlled by a complex regulatory system.

1. First, an electrical system controls the circulation and the conducting system of the heart. This is balanced between the vagus nerve and a number of sympathetic nerves. The vagus nerve slows your heart down and the sympathetic nerves speed your heart up. The overall control of these comes from your brain and allows your heart to slow down or speed up, your blood pressure to rise and fall, and the blood flow to different organs to be increased or decreased differentially. So, for example, after a meal blood is diverted to your intestines and away from your limb muscles. As a result you may get cramp and not be able to swim properly, hence the advice not to swim after a meal. Similarly, after a heavy meal you may get angina when you walk, as your heart is having to pump more blood to the digestive system to absorb the food, and the additional demand to pump blood to your leg muscles may give the heart a 'cramp' or angina.

2. Secondly, a hormonal system interacts with the electrical system. This includes the release of adrenaline and noradrenaline (called the sympathoadrenomedullary system) and cortisol (called the pituitaryadrenal cortical system). Other hormones such as renin, angiotensin and aldosterone are also released. These hormones respond to situations perceived by the body (for example fight, flight, despair, challenge, dehydration, etc.), usually in an appropriate way, but sometimes their release can be excessive, especially in response to emotions (*see below*).

The Effect of Emotions on the Cardiovascular System

Research shows that emotions profoundly affect the cardiovascular system. Blushing, pallor and fainting are familiar responses to an emotional situation. Emotions appear to trigger two main hormonal (neuroendocrine) responses.

Fight or Flight

The first of these hormonal responses is called 'the fight or flight reaction' and is associated with the release of adrenaline and noradrenaline. (This group of hormones is released by the sympathoadrenomedullary system.) It is crucially involved with situations that require attention or vigilance. If you are faced with an aggressive attack then noradrenaline is more important; if you are uncertain or anxious, both adrenaline and noradrenaline are involved. There is an increase in heart rate, blood pressure and in oxygen consumption in preparation. The result is to send more blood to the muscles ready for the challenge ahead. In addition glucose, uric acid and free fatty acids are released (all of which will provide an immediate energy source) and the blood tends to clot more quickly (which may be useful in a fight).

The fight or flight reaction was clearly important for our

prehistoric ancestors who had to face the challenge of, for example, attack by a wild animals. Corresponding challenges in today's Western world may be road rage, a confrontational argument, a stressful interview or mental arithmetic. They will still provoke the hormones of fight or flight, but the physical action will not be required. The glucose, fatty acids and increased clotting function of the blood which have been released are no longer needed for life-saving activity, and high levels in the blood can then affect the lining of the arteries. This is the precursor to atheroma (*see pages 77–9*). The increased tendency to clot may also be harmful as small arteries, like the coronary arteries, may become blocked.

Defeat and Despair

The second hormonal response to emotion is associated with release of cortisol through the pituitary-adrenal system. This response is linked with feelings of defeat, despair, loss and isolation.

These two systems are intimately linked and may be thought of as follows:

♦ Effort without distress is a joyous, happy state that is accompanied by adrenaline and noradrenaline secretion. Cortisol secretion is actively suppressed.

♦ Effort with distress (maybe associated with some of life's daily hassles) is accompanied by an increase in both adrenaline/noradrenaline and cortisol secretion.

♦ Distress without effort (such as giving up and feeling helpless) is accompanied by an outpouring of cortisol.

The Physical Consequences of Hormonal Activation

Our hormonal responses to our environment have evolved over many thousands of years. We still retain these responses, even though our environment has changed. Some people cope with these challenges better than others, maybe because they have adapted. However, anyone can be pushed beyond the limits of their endurance and tolerance and then they become much more reactive and sensitive to their hormonal outpourings.

The Psychological Effect of Hormonal Activation

You may feel anxious, as if you are 'on the run' from a tiger behind you. You may feel nervous or afraid of nothing in particular. Sometimes people cope with this by eating, drinking or smoking too much. You may become depressed and 'retreat from the tiger', resulting in isolation and more depression.

This can become a self-perpetuating cycle of fearing the fear until the triggers are recognised and revised. Finding what that trigger is and learning how to deal with it helps to quieten hormone activity (*see page 58*).

In this chapter we have been looking at the physical heart. In the next chapter we will see how closely it is linked with our emotional heart.

Chapter 4

ARTERIAL DISEASE, ANGINA, HEART ATTACKS AND HEART FAILURE

Heart disease presents a rich model for examining the relationship between lifestyle and health.
DEAN ORNISH

IN THIS CHAPTER we look at some of the most common forms of heart problems and explore some of the reasons why these illnesses may arise. Lifestyle factors and emotional health often play a major role.

Arterial Disease

The inner lining of your arteries should be smooth walled but, silently, over many years, a patchy deposit of fatty material is laid down. This is called atheroma. The build-up of atheroma causes arterial disease, which makes areas of the arteries narrower, thus reducing the amount of blood that can flow through them. Sometimes the fatty areas crack, leaving rough surfaces that cause red blood cells to stick to them and clot, a process called thrombosis. This may block the whole artery. Moreover the wall of the artery is weakened and may give way, causing bleeding (haemorrhage).

Atheroma causes:

♦ **Angina** when it narrows your coronary artery.

♦ **Heart attack** (also called a myocardial infarction or coronary thrombosis) when it blocks your coronary artery.

♦ **Stroke** (also called a CVA or cerebrovascular accident) when it blocks an artery to your brain.

♦ **Claudication** when it affects the arteries to your legs, causing pain and limping.

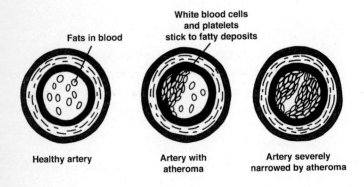

How Atheroma Develops

A normal coronary artery is smooth walled (left). *Atheroma narrows the artery* (centre) *and it eventually becomes very restrictive* (right).

Risk Factors for Atheroma

Many people think that atheroma is an inevitable consequence of getting old, but this is not so. Atheroma is more likely to occur if:

♦ You smoke.

♦ You have high blood pressure.

♦ It runs in your family.

♦ You have diabetes.

♦ You have high levels of cholesterol.

♦ You have certain lifestyle and personality characteristics (*see page 76*).

It is probably more likely to occur if you are overweight and take too little exercise.

What to Do

Clearly you can do a great deal to prevent the build-up of atheroma and thus reduce your chances of a heart attack or stroke.

It is very important that you do not smoke and that you take regular exercise. Eating sensibly and keeping your weight in check are also very important. These areas are discussed in more detail later (*see pages 219 and 220*).

It is well known that low-dose aspirin taken daily reduces the risk of angina, heart attacks and stroke in people with at least one risk factor and no history of cardiovascular disease. Always consult your doctor before taking aspirin, especially if you suffer from stomach ulcers or related problems or are on any other type of medication. Aspirin should only be taken with Warfarin when recommended by a doctor.

Angina

The word 'angina' is merely a descriptive term meaning 'chest pain'. The heart muscle (myocardium) is supplied by oxygen and other nutrients through the coronary arteries. When the heart works harder, during exercise or with excitement/ emotion, it requires more blood. If one or more of the arteries is narrowed due to atheroma, then there is an imbalance between what the heart muscle wants and what it gets. A warning pain develops and this pain is called angina. (There are other causes of angina such as severe aortic stenosis, or narrowed main outlet valve (aortic) *see page 117*, or hypertrophic cardiomyopathy – HOCM, or thick muscle disease, *see page 125*.)

Angina is generally felt as a tightness or a weight – usually not a sharp pain – on the chest, sometimes spreading to the shoulder, arm, neck or even jaw. One person described it as 'a giant crab clutching at my chest', another 'a terrible pressing sensation'. When the extra workload imposed on the heart is reduced, by resting for example, the pain disappears.

Angina is called chronic when it has been present for some time and is relatively predictable, occurring with certain activities or emotions. Angina can occur after meals (postprandial), at night (nocturnal) or sometimes at rest.

Angina is called unstable when there are frequent attacks of pain occurring without provocation. These often come and go in short periods of time. Unstable angina needs urgent treatment in hospital.

Risk Factors for Angina and Heart Attacks

The risk factors for angina are the same as for heart attacks. There are many risk factors but the following are considered the main independent risk factors.

Smoking
Smoking is a risk factor because the carbon monoxide in cigarettes joins the red pigment of the blood, called haemoglobin, and reduces its power to carry oxygen to the heart and other parts of the body. Nicotine stimulates the body to produce adrenaline, which makes the heart beat faster and raises the blood pressure. Both nicotine and carbon monoxide appear to make blood stickier, encouraging clotting or thrombosis.

The risk of heart disease rises with the amount smoked. In general, people who smoke have about twice as great a risk of heart attack as those who don't. In smokers under 50, heart attack death rates are up to 10 times greater than those of non-smokers of the same age.

Nowadays smoking is in decline, but this is not as marked in women as in men, possibly because smoking is perceived as a way to stay slim. Studies show that people who give up smoking after a heart attack live longer than those who don't, and stopping smoking is more effective than aspirin, clot-busters and beta blockers. It cuts death rates by a whacking 61 per cent. Unfortunately smoking is so addictive that even a brush with death is not enough to stop everyone.

High Blood Pressure

High blood pressure, or hypertension, makes the heart work harder and makes the left pump (ventricle) thicken or become hypertrophic (the medical term meaning 'thickening'). Death from heart disease is two to four times higher when the left ventricle is thickened.

In many cases high blood pressure is found during a routine examination, and when there are no symptoms it is often difficult to appreciate the value of taking tablets to lower the blood pressure. This does, however, have outstanding long-term benefits. The management of high blood pressure is discussed in more detail in the following chapter.

Family History

If you have a mother or father who died of a heart attack before they reached 60, you are five times more likely to have a fatal heart attack yourself than those who haven't. It may not just be heredity – family behaviour can make your risk worse. Family members can influence each other through passing on habits such as taking no exercise, eating a fatty diet and smoking.

If heart disease runs in your family, you can still lower your risk. Watching your weight and diet, having your cholesterol and blood pressure checked and taking regular exercise will be particularly helpful.

Diabetes

Diabetes is a disorder of the mechanism that converts the sugar in the blood into energy. The process requires the hormone insulin, which is produced by the pancreas after a meal. Diabetes which starts at a young age is nearly always treated with insulin. Diabetes which starts in later life is often treated with tablets. This second type of diabetes appears to be increasing, probably because of increased obesity, reduced activity and longer life expectancy.

High blood sugar attacks the small arteries of the body, including those of the heart. In diabetes it is often another blood fat, triglyceride, which is elevated and needs treating. A group of tablets called the fibrates are particularly useful when triglycerides are raised.

The rate of heart disease in diabetics is about three times that of the general population. This particularly applies to the late-onset form of diabetes. Diabetes is also a stronger risk factor for women than for men. A very important new study (the Hope Study) has shown that diabetics with one other risk factor for heart disease should take an ACE inhibitor (Ramipril), as this improves survival.

High Cholesterol

Fats ingested into the body are utilised by the tissues for cell processes. Any excess fats circulate around the body in the bloodstream as a type of cholesterol called low-density lipoprotein (LDL). Total body cholesterol is made up of LDL and HDL (high-density lipoprotein). It is a high level of LDL which contributes to heart disease, together with triglycerides. On the other hand high levels of HDL (the 'good' cholesterol) have a preventative role in heart disease.

Total cholesterol (made up of HDL and LDL) is usually measured after fasting for 12 hours and in the general population should be below 6.5umol/L. In people with heart disease, a reduction to below 5.0 or less, with emphasis on a lower LDL portion, is the aim. This can be achieved by diet, but often tablets are required.

One in 500 people inherits a condition called familial hypercholesterolaemia, where the blood cholesterol levels are virtually double the norm. This usually needs medication.

Social Isolation and Loneliness

This appears to be particularly relevant when established social support structures are lost – after moving, for example. It is a risk factor independent of all the other factors listed and is significantly associated with a high risk of heart attack and sudden death. Ensuring good social support has improved the outlook in patients with heart disease.

Control and Job Strain

Work situations involving high demand but low control appear to have a significant influence on the development of angina, heart attacks and high blood pressure. This is in contrast to those for whom a high demand is associated with a high degree of control.

Understanding your own position may help you approach this difficult area of your working life. While it is often thought that it is the overworking male executive who is most prone to a heart attack, it is often those doing clerical jobs or boring repetitive ones who are more at risk. The most important thing seems to be control of the time schedule. (For more on stress, *see* Chapter 3.)

Loss of Well-being (Life Event Stress)

Life changes that deprive individuals of important sources of emotional security, self-esteem or a sense of identity are likely to be followed by a higher than normal risk of angina, heart attack and death.

A classic study looked at widowers in the years after the death of their wives. In the first six months a 40 per cent higher death rate was found in this group compared to the expected death rate in the same age range, and 67 per cent of this was due to heart disease.

A controlled trial involving the treatment of people with psychological intervention after heart attacks has shown a 47 per cent decline in death in the treated group compared to the non-treated group.

Angry and Hostile Behaviour

Angry and hostile behaviour has been found to be an independent risk factor of the same order of magnitude as blood pressure, smoking and high cholesterol.

Most people have heard about Type A behaviour. This is discussed in more detail on page 143, but initially was thought to represent dynamic, high-achieving people. The important components of Type A behaviour have now been honed down to anger (which is frequently hidden) and hostility – especially when a situation threatens the person with a perceived loss of control over their surroundings. Recalling an incident that provoked real anger has been used during a catheter test (the X-ray study that is used to look at the coronary arteries) and this revealed further marked narrowing in diseased coronary arteries.

Phobic Anxiety

People with phobic anxiety feel anxious in certain situations, but if these situations are avoided they do not feel anxious. A recent study in London asked about common phobias, such as fear of enclosed spaces, going out alone, illness, heights and crowds, and found that they were strongly related to subsequent angina, heart attacks and death from heart disease, but not to deaths from other causes. (It is important to note that this study showed specifically that existing heart disease did not in itself lead to heightened phobic anxiety.) The postulated mechanism included hyperventilation (overbreathing, *see page 58*) and an exaggerated response of cortisol, adrenaline and noradrenaline (*see page 74*).

Depression

Major depression increases the risk of heart disease substantially and after a heart attack there is a five-fold greater risk of death in people who remain or who become depressed. People who have mild depression (but who don't fulfil medical criteria for a major depression) have a twofold increase in risk of heart attack.

The mechanism again appears to be increased activation of the pituitary-adrenal axis leading to increased cortisol secretion. Psychological therapies and drugs can both be very helpful.

Sedentary Lifestyle

A major risk factor in industrialised societies is a sedentary lifestyle that, if corrected, could have the greatest impact on the prevention of heart disease. The less physical activity you do, the more likely you are to get heart disease. Moreover, exercise and diet after heart attacks may prevent the progression of disease and further attacks.

Walking for 40 minutes three times a week has been shown to improve the cardiovascular status of 70-year-olds to that of 50-year-olds. The US Surgeon General has stated that every adult should accumulate 30 minutes or more of moderately intense physical activity, preferably every day of the week.

Diet

Most people living in Western societies eat too many calories and consume an unbalanced diet. Certain foods can be eaten more freely than others – vegetables, fruit, carbohydrates (potato, rice, pasta and bread) and fish. Don't give up meat if it means you just eat more cheese sauce on your vegetables; some meat is fine. Just eat a little less of everything. A certain amount of alcohol seems good but, like everything, too much does affect the heart directly. Also, alcohol puts on the calories. Over a third of British women and a quarter of British men are seriously overweight. Being fat is linked with higher cholesterol and higher blood pressure and you may not be able to exercise or even move at a normal pace. The moderately overweight are 80 per cent more at risk of heart disease than leaner people. For more on diet, *see pages 220–1*.

Other Risk Factors

Less is known about the following risk factors.

Homocysteine Levels

An elevated level of homocysteine, a blood protein, is more common in people with heart disease than in those who do not have it. There is also a specific family-linked version, familial homocysteinaemia, which predisposes to premature coronary artery disease.

Homocysteine induces an accelerated progression of atheroma, but the mechanism behind this is not yet clear. It may be related to an interaction with fibrinogen, which is part of the clotting process (*see below*).

Homocysteine levels seem to be higher in women than in men, and it may be relevant to screen women with heart disease (but a normal cholesterol profile) for raised homocysteine.

Fibrinogen and Clotting Factors

Fibrinogen is part of the clotting system in the blood. Some people have higher levels and this is a strong predictor of subsequent heart disease in otherwise healthy people, and of further heart attacks in people with established heart disease.

At the moment, fibrinogen is not routinely measured as a risk factor as it is not known whether it is related to the disease process, or if it is just a marker of the activity and progression of atheroma build-up.

What You Can Do to Lower the Risks

If you have any of the risk factors discussed above, there are several simple measures you can take to decrease your risk of angina and heart attack.

If the cholesterol is found to be elevated in your blood, try to decrease your saturated fat intake. Saturated fat is found in animal fats – the fat on meat and in butter and hard cheese. Transfats should also be avoided. These are the hydrogenated fats found in hard margarines and a lot of cakes, biscuits, pastries and takeaway food. Try to use fats high in mono-unsaturated fats, such as olive oil and rapeseed oil, and spreads containing polyunsaturated oil.

Margarine spreads capable of reducing cholesterol concentrations are now available in the UK. Bencol contains stanol esters derived from wood pulp which reduce the amount of cholesterol absorbed by the gut. Pro-Vita Flora is another spread that appears to lower cholesterol. A recent study in Finland, where people consumed 3 g of Benecol per day – equivalent to generously spreading three pieces of toast with the margarine – showed that total cholesterol concentrations can be lowered by up to 10 per cent and LDL (the bad cholesterol) may be lowered by up to 14 per cent if it is eaten as part of a low-fat low-cholesterol diet. It does not appear to make any appreciable difference to concentrations of triglycerides or HDL (the good cholesterol). It may increase bowel frequency. Recent reports in the press have suggested that the spread may not have the results suggested by the makers, but it does seem effective when assessed in trials if it is used in the quantities suggested by the manufacturers.

Another helpful fact is that taking folic acid lowers the level of homocysteine. Thus the best defence against high homocysteine levels appears to be an increased consumption of foods high in folic acid, such as vegetables and fortified grain products. Alternatively, take a folic acid supplement daily.

Simple measures to increase exercise can also be quite effective.

♦ Don't take the lift to go up two floors – walk up instead.

♦ Park the car in a safe place but not too close to work and walk the rest of the way.

Stopping smoking is always helpful. For more on this, *see page 223*.

Treatment for Angina

Self-help
Someone with angina can often help themselves a great deal by learning to listen to their heart (*see pages 15–18*), so that they can cope with the limitations the condition imposes on them.

Drug Treatment

♦ Everyone who has angina should be taking a baby (paediatric) dose of aspirin – 75 mg – which acts on the platelets in the blood and so makes it clot less quickly. Aspirin should be taken with food, since it can irritate the stomach lining.

♦ Most people will also need a tablet to lower their cholesterol. The most common type is a statin, which not only lowers cholesterol but also appears to stabilise the fatty areas of narrowing, or plaque, in the coronary arteries.

♦ The simplest form of treatment is a tablet or spray under the tongue called GTN (glyceryl trinitrate). This acts by dilating the arteries and veins, thus allowing more blood to reach the heart. Sometimes GTN is associated with headaches. It is used either when you get an angina attack or before doing an activity which usually provokes angina. There are longer-acting forms of GTN called nitrates, which can be taken in tablet form or via a skin patch.

♦ Beta blockers are often prescribed for people with angina since they slow the heart down and thus allow more activity to occur before the heart rate reaches the speed at which not enough blood can get to the heart muscle. Beta blockers are not usually prescribed if you have asthma, intermittent claudication (pain in the legs due to narrowed leg arteries as a result of atheroma) or insulin-dependent diabetes, as they can mask the effects of a hypoglycaemic attack. They can lead to some side-effects, such as impotence.

♦ Calcium antagonists may be prescribed to people if they cannot take beta blockers. These drugs dilate the arteries by relaxing the smooth muscle in the wall of the artery. Diltiazem is usually used because it also slows the heart down. Sometimes other calcium antagonists are added to beta blockers for an additional effect – Nifedipine and Amlodipine are examples. All these tablets may make the ankles swell a little.

♦ Potassium channel blockers are a newer class of medication which work by dilating the arteries to the heart by blocking the potassium channel of the smooth muscle. An example is Nicorandil. It can sometimes give headaches.

Surgery
Treatment for angina may involve surgery – coronary (balloon) angioplasty or coronary artery bypass grafting (CABG) (*see page 185*). Such treatments are effective in relieving the anginal pain and allow a person to do much more than before. They improve the situation but do not take away the underlying problem.

Other Treatments
When alterations in lifestyle, and medication, angioplasty and bypass grafting, have not alleviated the symptoms of angina, other treatments can include any of the following:

♦ Sometimes a TENS machine can reduce the perception of pain, as can hypnosis and self-hypnosis, and careful self-management of the balance of rest and effort can make the pain feel less acute.

♦ Laser treatment to the lining of the heart may be possible (percutaneous myocardial revasculariation, or PMR).

♦ Treatment can sometimes be possible with blocking nerves in the neck (stellate ganglion block), or spinal cord stimulation.

Heart Attacks

A heart attack occurs when a coronary artery becomes blocked by a blood clot, usually (but not always) at the site of a narrowing; the result is that the heart muscle does not get its blood supply. Pain develops which, unlike angina, does not cease after a few minutes' rest. Part of the heart muscle is damaged irreparably (called a myocardial infarction, or MI) and the heart pump does not function as well.

New treatments are now aimed at giving an injection to dissolve (lyse) the clot and thus save or limit the amount of heart muscle damage. This is called coronary thrombolysis. To be most effective the injection needs to be given within six hours of the start of the pain, but it can still be helpful for quite a lot longer.

If the heart muscle is damaged beyond repair, it is replaced by scar tissue. The heart does have good reserve capacity and after recovery from the heart attack the loss of a small part of the heart muscle may not interfere with the ability to return to a normal lifestyle.

The area of heart muscle damaged is referred to by doctors by position. This could be the undersurface or inferior part; the front surface or anterior; the back surface or posterior. So if you hear someone described as having had 'an inferior MI', this means that the heart attack has damaged the undersurface of the heart and not that it is of a lower or lesser type.

A heart attack can be complicated by rhythm disturbances, or arrhythmias. The most serious of these is when the ventricle or heart pump starts to quiver very fast in an uncoordinated way and no useful heartbeat occurs. This is called ventricular fibrillation. It can sometimes be stopped with a thump to the chest wall but usually needs an electrical shock (DC cardioversion). It is this rhythm disturbance that is responsible for most of the deaths associated with heart attacks and it usually occurs soon after the attack starts. It is important to get to a coronary care unit or specialised ambulance quickly. Heart attacks are a medical emergency.

Risk Factors for Heart Attack

The lifetime risk of coronary heart disease – angina, heart attacks or death – at the age of 40 is 1:2 for men and 1:3 for women, according to US researchers. The lifetime risk does fall with age, but even at 70, 1:3 men and 1:4 women will be expected to have a heart-related event.

As the risk factors for heart attacks also pertain to angina, they have been described more fully above (*see pages 80–6*). In brief, some of the risk factors are:

♦ Smoking

♦ High blood pressure

♦ Family history

♦ Diabetes

♦ High levels of cholesterol

♦ Certain lifestyle and personality characteristics (for example depression, job strain, isolation, angry/hostile personality).

Trigger Factors for Heart Attacks

Heart attacks are more likely to occur within the first three hours of waking (irrespective of the time of waking) than at other times of the day. This is probably due to the fact that on wakening, heart rate, blood pressure, adrenaline/noradrenaline release and platelet stickiness are all increased. In addition, the body's ability to decrease clotting is at its lowest first thing in the morning.

Trigger factors such as exercise, cold and mental stress all probably work through increasing the heart rate, blood pressure, adrenaline/noradrenaline and cortisol, platelet stickiness and clotting activity.

What to Do in the Event of a Heart Attack

Although the pain of a heart attack can be similar to angina, it will not go away after rest or GTN (tablets or spray under the tongue that dilates coronary arteries). If after three doses of GTN taken three minutes apart the pain is not improving or is getting worse, you should seek help. Chew an aspirin while waiting. (*See page 244.*)

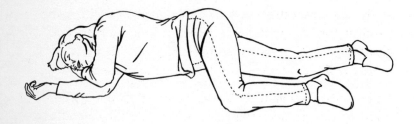

The Recovery Position
If you are with someone who has just had a heart attack, turn them on their side with the arms positioned as shown. The underneath leg should be straight and the other leg should be bent across it.

Treatment Following a Heart Attack

There are many things that you can do to help yourself following a heart attack (*see pages 244–5*). In addition:

- Most people will be prescribed aspirin and have a statin for their cholesterol (*see* 'Treatment for Angina', *page 88*).

- Beta blockers and ACE inhibitors have been shown to improve survival after a heart attack, so many people will be taking these, sometimes just for six months and sometimes for longer.

- Warfarin is sometimes prescribed if a blood clot has been found in the cavity of the heart pump (left ventricle) and is usually continued for six months.

Heart Failure

Heart failure is not as frightening as it sounds. It does not mean that your heart is about to stop. It is a term used to describe a condition where the heart is not pumping adequately. It is, nevertheless, a serious condition. A recent study found that there was only about a 60 per cent chance of survival for 18 months from first diagnosis (although this clearly depends on the cause and varies considerably).

The most common symptoms of heart failure are:

- Shortness of breath. This may be most common when you are doing physical exercise such as walking or climbing upstairs or when you are lying in bed. You may find you need an increasing number of pillows to enable you to breathe when in bed. Sometimes you may wake in the middle of the night because you are having difficulty in breathing.

- Swollen feet, ankles and legs due to a build-up of fluid. This is called oedema.

- Reduced exercise tolerance.

- Tiredness or weakness.

- Distended abdomen and poor appetite.

- Irregular heartbeats.

The Causes of Heart Failure

Heart failure may be the result of heart attacks damaging the heart muscle; or the strain or stretch of the heart pump because a valve is narrowed or leaking; or a disease that has directly weakened the heart muscle – a condition which is called cardiomyopathy. Cardiomyopathy can be the result of a viral or other infection, or can sometimes be inherited. Prolonged and poorly controlled high blood pressure can also lead to stretching of the heart muscle and thus heart failure.

All of these enlarge the pumping chambers of the heart (the ventricles). This can affect either the left ventricle (more common), the right ventricle or both. The ventricles then become very large and sluggish.

Coping with Heart Failure

Heart failure can be a frightening and frustrating condition, but many of the coping strategies described in this book will be helpful.

Restricting salt intake (which encourages fluid to be retained) and fluid intake (on the advice of your doctor or nurse) can be very useful. Certain tablets, such as non-steroidal anti-inflammatories (e.g. ibuprufen) taken for arthritis can predispose you to accumulating fluid and should be avoided if possible.

You should take as much regular exercise as you feel able to do. One of your body's responses to heart failure is loss of muscle bulk, especially in the legs, and if you increase your muscle strength, especially in the legs, you will improve the amount of exercise you can do and may decrease your symptoms. Even when sitting in a chair you can practise exercises – lifting a weighted bag with a straight leg, for example.

Drug Treatment for Heart Failure

In heart failure the heart is usually enlarged. If you imagine a large village pond, there are often quiet still areas around the edge where water does not move as quickly. The same is true in a large heart and in these areas small clots may develop which could be harmful. Aspirin reduces the tendency to clot formation and is protective, so it is often prescribed.

Diuretics such as Frusemide (Furosemide), Bumetanide and Thiazides are used, as they increase the amount of water expelled from the body by the kidneys. These tablets improve the breathlessness of heart failure as they help remove fluid that has accumulated on the lungs. They will also reduce the swelling of the legs, ankles and abdomen.

Potassium-saving diuretics such as Spironolactone, which affect the hormone system of the kidneys, have recently been shown to be of major benefit in heart failure as well as helping to relieve the fluid accumulation.

ACE inhibitors are a group of tablets that affect an enzyme in the blood. They help to relieve breathlessness and have been shown to have long-term benefit on the way the heart muscle pumps. In 20 per cent of people (most commonly women) they can cause a cough, so that a slightly different tablet, called an ACE 2 antagonist, may be given. It is now thought that the combining of these tablets may be helpful for heart failure, especially in diabetics.

Until recently beta blockers were not prescribed for heart failure, but it has been shown that when the symptoms of heart failure have been treated with diuretics and ACE inhibitors, the addition of small doses of beta blockers really improves the long-term outlook. Studies have shown considerably fewer admissions to hospital with fluid overload, and longer survival. Tablets such as Bisoprolol, Carvedilol or Metoprolol may be started at very low doses and slowly increased.

Warfarin may be given if the heart is very enlarged to prevent clots forming in the cavity of the heart. Warfarin slows down the clot formation in the body. In overdosage it causes massive bleeding and hence is used as a poison in small animals, but the level of Warfarin dosage in humans is carefully controlled.

Rhythm disturbance tablets may also be required as the enlarged heart may be prone to fast abnormal rhythms. Sometimes pacemakers can also help if they stimulate both ventricles ('biventricular pacing').

Chapter 5

HIGH BLOOD PRESSURE

The heart has its reasons which reason knows nothing of.
BLAISE PASCAL, *Pensées*

HIGH BLOOD PRESSURE is a common condition which affects between one in five and one in ten of the population. Yet despite its frequent occurrence, in 90 per cent of cases no underlying cause for the condition can be found. The role of stress, it has been argued, is an important factor, so coming to terms with your emotional response to stress will be crucial in managing high blood pressure.

Each time the heart's pump (ventricle) pushes blood out, it creates a surge of pressure to distribute the blood around the system to the organs. The peak of this pressure is called systolic pressure. The baseline level to which the pressure falls back after the surge created by the contraction of the heart muscle is called diastolic pressure. A typical reading might be 120 systolic and 80 diastolic, recorded as 120/80. The figures are measured from a column of mercury measured in millimetres (mm). When your blood pressure is found to be above 145/95 on a number of occasions it is considered to be elevated. Sometimes only the systolic (top figure) is elevated; this is called systolic hypertension. Occasionally only the diastolic (bottom figure) is elevated; this is called diastolic hypertension.

There is also a phenomenon called 'white coat hypertension', when the blood pressure is quite elevated when taken by a doctor. That is why blood pressure is usually taken on a number of occasions to try and obtain a realistic reading. An ambulatory blood pressure recording can be helpful – this is where a blood pressure cuff is applied to the arm and inflated automatically three times every hour. The result is recorded on a cassette attached to a belt worn around the waist. It shows the blood pressure taken over a 24-hour period, removes the stress of going to the clinic and allows an assessment of what is the more normal blood pressure. There has been some work, however, which suggests that people with white coat hypertension are more reactive in general and may in fact go on to develop high blood pressure.

Most people with high blood pressure have no symptoms. Headaches usually only occur if the pressure is very high and they are more likely to be due to other causes such as anxiety. Because high blood pressure occurs without symptoms it is a condition that can only be detected by measuring and thus it is important, especially with increasing age, to have your blood pressure measured regularly, especially if people in your family have high blood pressure.

Studies have shown that people with diabetes are more susceptible to the effect of blood pressure; thus while in a non-diabetic the optimum blood pressure might be 140/90, in diabetics the optimum is 135/80. The combination of diabetes and high blood pressure on the heart, kidneys, brain and eyes is particularly harmful, so every effort is made to check the blood pressure frequently.

Untreated high blood pressure does predispose you to a much greater risk of developing strokes, heart attacks, angina, heart failure and kidney disease. But regular blood pressure measurement and treatment are effective in reducing this risk.

The Causes of High Blood Pressure

As stated earlier, in 90 per cent of cases no underlying cause for high blood pressure can be found. This is called essential hypertension. On rare occasions, causes such as narrowing of an artery to the kidney, overproduction of a hormone from the adrenal gland, or some forms of severe kidney disease are found. Just occasionally some tablets can cause the blood pressure to be raised, for example those used to treat ulcers, arthritis or depression.

The oral contraceptive pill increases the blood pressure in a small proportion of women, so it is important to have your blood pressure checked regularly when taking the pill.

Even if you have high blood pressure you should be able to have a baby without risk, although extra supervision is required. High blood pressure may sometimes develop for the first time in pregnancy (pre-eclampsia) and it may require treatment with bed rest or drugs, especially in the weeks before delivery. Blood pressure usually returns to normal after the baby is delivered.

Risk Factors for High Blood Pressure

Weight

High blood pressure is very common in overweight people and losing a few kilograms often reduces blood pressure. For every kilogram of weight lost the blood pressure is said to fall by 4 mm mercury.

Alcohol

Heavy drinking definitely raises your blood pressure. The general guidelines are no more than 14–21 units per week for women and 21–28 units per week for men. If you stick to these limits, your drinking is unlikely to be associated with increased blood pressure. Remember, 1 unit is half a pint of beer, a glass of wine or a single measure of spirits.

Salt

The role of a high-salt diet in the development of high blood pressure has been increasingly found to be of importance. Do not add salt to the food on your plate and reduce or omit it when cooking. Also avoid foods with a high salt content, especially pre-prepared/ready-to-cook foods or ham. Check the labels carefully. Flavour food with spices instead. A recent study (*Dietary Approaches to Stop Hypertension: 'DASH'*) showed marked reductions in blood pressure in both men and women and in people from all ethnic backgrounds when salt intake was reduced.

Stress

The role of stress in the development of essential hypertension has been hotly debated for many years but hurry, worry and anger have long been put forward as important antecedents for the development of high blood pressure. Strenuous exercise or anxiety both raise the blood pressure as a normal response. This is part of the preparation for 'fight or flight'. What is increasingly clear is that there are individuals who are more reactive to such stimuli than others and that repeated surges of blood pressure arising from the exposure to stresses can cause structural changes in the walls of the arteries. In turn this causes an increase in the resistance put up by the body, so that the heart has to raise its pumping pressure to overcome this. The normal level of blood pressure is then reset at a higher level.

Unlike coronary artery disease, a diagnosis of high blood pressure has not been shown to be preceded by stressful life events but by a greater association with prolonged and chronic environmental stress. For example, air traffic controllers, who are engaged in a taxing operation that requires constant alertness and carries heavy responsibilities, were shown to have a rate of high blood pressure four times that of second-class airmen. They were also more likely to develop high blood pressure at an early age.

Job responsibility and educational achievement have also emerged as important factors in high blood pressure – particularly the discrepancy between them. For example, individuals who had achieved a high social and occupational position but had little formal education tend to have higher blood pressure than individuals in whom the discrepancy is much less.

Family History

People with normal blood pressure but who have family members with high blood pressure have been shown to have exaggerated and prolonged responses to anxiety and other emotional stressors and they may also retain more fluid and sodium. High blood pressure does seem to run in some families.

Ethnic Origin

Studies have shown that high blood pressure (and diabetes) is raised two to threefold in Southeast Asians, Caribbeans and West Africans living in Britain. People of African descent are not more susceptible in general to high blood pressure, so lifestyle factors are probably responsible. These may include a higher salt intake, a greater tendency to increased weight and other day-to-day stresses.

Personality Profile

It has been noted that people with high blood pressure demonstrate a desire to please and a wish to be liked, but while outwardly calm, their internal stance is one of suppressed anger, tension, suspicion and hostility. Thus the person with high blood pressure is thought to struggle with an accumulation of anger and resentment that they are unable to resolve; this affects the nervous system and results in the resetting of the blood pressure at a higher level.

Treatment of High Blood Pressure

Nowhere perhaps is the effect of the mind on the cardiovascular system so powerfully seen as in the treatment of hypertension. The placebo effect and the therapeutic expectation of the patient can provoke dramatic short-term responses. The efficacy of treatment is thus difficult to assess, but certainly some psychological techniques have been shown to be effective in producing a long-term reduction in blood pressure. Such techniques include progressive muscle relaxation, biofeedback and meditation.

Medication may include Thiazide diuretics, beta blockers, ACE inhibitors or ACE2 antagonists, calcium antagonists and alpha blockers, as well as many other drugs. It sometimes takes a little time to find the right tablets for each person and it may be that a combination of tablets is best. Sometimes ambulatory blood pressure monitoring (blood pressure recorded through the day on a monitor attached around the waist) can help to assess the treatment response. If you have side-effects from one of your tablets you should discuss them with your doctor, as there are many different effective medications to choose from.

Sometimes in response to certain drugs the blood pressure may become too low and the tablets will need to be reduced. Symptoms of low blood pressure include dizziness and light-headedness. Low blood pressure in an otherwise normal individual is not a cause for concern. In the UK it is not treated, although this is not the case in some other European countries.

Managing High Blood Pressure

> It is essential to control high blood pressure.

The goal for people who have had a heart attack is to maintain their blood pressure at under 140/85. The goal for people with diabetes is 130/80.

If you have high blood pressure, have a full discussion with your doctor about recommended medication. Then, put your own self-help into operation.

♦ Watch your weight.

♦ Watch your alcohol and salt intake.

♦ Start a good cardiac exercise programme where you gradually stretch your exercise tolerance. Exercise is hugely beneficial – for weight management, joint and muscle stretching, lung capacity, a growing sense of confidence and well-being and also for help with depression. Swimming, aerobics or vigorous walking are all good examples.

♦ Watch your stress levels and really take reducing your responses to stressors seriously. We cannot change the world or the government overnight, but we can change our response to whatever we allow to irritate us in our private worlds.

♦ Know in advance exactly what experiences put your blood pressure at risk of being raised. If those situations are unavoidable – moving house, a demanding job, rebellious teenagers – plan to become a very good manager. Plan your approach as a conqueror, not a victim. Learn some techniques that give you a licence to stop your activities for five minutes. This may be by relaxed breathing, autohypnosis or meditation. Situations that cause hurry, worry and anger may be offset by five minutes of biofeedback.

● VISUALISATION TO REGULATE YOUR BLOOD PRESSURE

The following exercise was generously given to us for this book by psychotherapist Susie Nixon, who has had many years experience of working with heart patients. She suggests using the following exercise each day while you are settling your blood pressure to an acceptable level.

● Find a comfortable place to sit or lie down.

● Take some time to rest and relax your body. Close your eyes. Allow your breathing to become slow and regular. Each out-breath makes you feel more relaxed and at peace.

● Now imagine that you are in a beautiful garden. It may be a garden you know or a garden that comes to you now in your imagination. Walk around this garden. Notice its flowers, shrubs, trees, sounds, smells, and the sun and blue sky above.

● In this garden there is a house. This house is the house of your body and mind. Enter this house and walk the corridors until you find the control room.

● Go into the room and you will find and see your pulse and blood pressure dials. Turn the dials to the numbers you would like.

● Know that you are in charge and in control.

● Gradually become aware of your surroundings. Feel where you are sitting or lying. Remain another few minutes in your relaxed state. When ready, open your eyes.

● Note how well and relaxed you feel.

The following exercise is also included on page 231, but has a particular influence on steadying bloody pressure.

● THE HOUSE OF HEART VISUALISATION

Again, find a comfortable place to sit or lie. Close your eyes. Take time to relax your body. Allow your breathing to become slow and regular.

Now imagine yourself standing in a meadow – with blue sky and sun overhead.

It is summer. Notice the atmosphere and feeling of the meadow – its sights, sounds and smells. In the meadow you find a special house. This house represents you. Notice what it is made of and how it looks.

When you are ready, enter the house. Walk into the hall and you notice a number of rooms.

In one room you will hear a rhythmic pounding and you will know that this is the room representing your heart. Enter this room. Take a good look around.

If there is anything in the room that seems out of sorts, disconnected, dark or unhealthy, go towards this part of the room and place your own healing hands upon it. As you are doing this, ask:

'What does my heart most need?'

'What is it that I am doing and my heart does not like?'

'If you could speak, heart, what would you say?'

As you stay with what emerges in this visualisation, become aware of your own capacity for healing and for holding the wisdom of your own heart. Believe in this natural wisdom and knowing.

Chapter 6

PALPITATIONS

And then my heart with pleasure fills and dances with the daffodils.

WILLIAM WORDSWORTH

PALPITATIONS ARE WHEN your heart beats in an unusual fashion. They may be extra beats or fast, regular or irregular beats, or sometimes very slow beats.

Extra Beats (Premature Beats or Ectopics)

Ectopic beats are one of the commonest forms of palpitation. These are experienced as an early beat in your heart's regular sequence, followed by a pause and then a more forceful beat. You are often likely to feel them at night, especially when lying on your left side, or when sitting quietly or immediately after exercise. In nearly all cases they should not cause concern and no treatment is indicated.

Sometimes excess caffeine or alcohol can predispose some people to have more ectopic beats. There is also no doubt that they cause anxiety in some people and this may also exacerbate them. Relaxation techniques can be very helpful. Occasionally small doses of medication are given if they are really troublesome. In individuals who are otherwise healthy they rarely indicate any underlying problems.

In people with coronary artery disease (angina, heart attacks) ectopic beats can arise from the area of scar tissue. It is not normally necessary to take tablets to suppress them; treating them does not seem to affect the outcome and the side-effects of medication are therefore not worthwhile. Such ectopics may come and go.

Careful studies have shown that there is a definite association between an increase in ectopic beats and emotional stress, such as driving a car in heavy traffic or watching a football game. They can be reduced in some people by biofeedback and muscle relaxation techniques.

Tachycardia (Fast Heartbeat)

Sinus Tachycardia

All of us will have experienced occasions when our heart has raced, usually because of an anxious or emotional experience. The heartbeat starts slowly, gets faster and then gradually declines in speed. Sometimes these fast heartbeats become disproportionate to the situation and may become part of a phobic response. Heart rates exceeding 140 beats per minute have been documented in normal people driving in heavy London traffic or speaking at medical meetings. Although sinus tachycardia can be uncomfortable, it does not indicate underlying problems.

Atrial Fibrillation

This is the most common type of palpitation. The irregular beats are caused by disorganisation of the initiation of the heartbeat in the atrium (receiving chamber). Usually they are fast and irregular. Some people are unaware of having them, whereas others can get rapid uncomfortable heartbeats. Because the heart is no longer beating in an orderly way it is less efficient and you may experience fatigue, breathlessness and reduction in exercise tolerance. Sometimes the symptoms are confused with those of depression (as fatigue and lethargy are common to both) until investigations are carried out.

The Causes of Atrial Fibrillation

Some people suffer from atrial fibrillation after excessive alcohol or a viral infection. Others get the palpitations inter-mittently (lasting from seconds to weeks) over many years. These are labelled 'paroxysmal'. In these instances the heart is often structurally normal.

In other cases atrial fibrillation becomes the established rhythm of the heart. This may occur due to an overactive thyroid, mitral stenosis (narrowed mitral or inlet valve to the left ventricle) or past rheumatic fever, but in many cases it is the result of coronary heart disease or high blood pressure.

Treatment of Atrial Fibrillation

When the irregularity has only been present a short while, it is usual for your doctor to try and get the heart to return to regular beating, either by tablets alone or in combination with electric shock treatment.

The proper name for electric shock treatment is DC (direct current) cardioversion. It is unfortunate that the term has overtones of the electric shock therapy used in some forms of depression (electroconvulsive therapy). Nevertheless, it is an excellent form of treatment which aims to disrupt the little waves of fibrillation and allow the SA node to re-establish the dominant role as the pacesetter. It is done on an out-patient basis under a short-acting general anaesthetic. Once under the anaesthetic a paddle is placed on the front of the chest and another either at the side or at the back. Usually a low voltage of direct current is used to start with.

This is increased to higher voltages if the heart does not return to regular beating.

You will have started taking Warfarin at least six weeks before the cardioversion and then continue on it for at least a month afterwards. Sometimes additional tablets may be given to better prepare the heart to return to regular beating. The treatment is usually successful, although not in every case. The shorter the time that the atrial fibrillation has been present and the more normal the underlying heart structure is, the better the chance of converting to a regular rhythm. Afterwards you will probably be given some hydrocortisone cream to apply to the chest where the paddles had been placed, as this area can sometimes be a little sore.

If DC cardioversion does not succeed or the irregularity has been present for some time, the rapid heartbeats of atrial fibrillation are controlled with tablets such as digoxin, beta blockers or amiodarone. To prevent you from going back into atrial fibrillation after the electrical shock therapy or if you have intermittent atrial fibrillation you may be prescribed tablets such as flecainide, verapamil, sotalol and propafenone.

Anti-coagulant Treatment – Warfarin and Aspirin

With atrial fibrillation, the atrium or collecting chamber of the heart no longer empties all the blood within it, so little backwaters of blood form where flow is sluggish. Blood clots can develop in these areas so in many cases blood-thinning agents such as aspirin or Warfarin are used to try and prevent little blood clots from leaving the heart and circulating around the body, and possibly causing strokes.

Supraventricular Tachycardias (SVT)

These are fast heartbeats often occurring at rates between 160 and 220 beats per minute. They usually start and stop suddenly. Supraventricular tachycardias start in the top part of the heart and are sometimes due to a sort of race-track developing in the atrium (receiving chamber), around which the electrical impulse careers rapidly.

● SELF-HELP FOR SUPRAVENTRICULAR TACHYCARDIAS

● **The valsalva manoeuvre** Take a breath in and try and push the breath out but without letting any air out of your nose or mouth (rather like trying to strain to pass a motion or to 'bear down' during labour).

● **Diving reflex** Immersing the whole face in a basin of cold water can stop these palpitations. This is especially helpful in young children – a five-second immersion should be adequate. Sucking ice can also be very effective.

● **Carotid sinus massage** If you turn your head towards your shoulder and feel for the angle of the jaw, just behind this and in front of your ear you will find a big muscle which travels down towards your collar-bone. Follow the edge of this muscle downwards, and about halfway you will feel an arterial pulsation. This is the carotid pulse. If you slowly massage the pulse, the palpitations may stop.

Some people are very aware that stressful situations may provoke their supraventricular tachycardias. Learning about the situations that are associated with your SVT may be very helpful.

Treatment for Supraventricular Tachycardias

In many cases tablets are required, such as sotalol, flecainide, amiodarone, propafenone, verapamil and diltiazem. These will be prescribed by your doctor.

In some instances the race-track can be blocked with a high-energy shock delivered by a wire inserted temporarily into the heart from the leg (a technique called ablation). The ablation treatment is done in hospital and you may be there for 24 hours or so. This treatment is often reserved for SVTs which do not subside with tablets, although it is the treatment of choice for certain types of SVT (such as Wolf Parkinson White syndrome) which have well-described race-tracks.

ZOË

Zoë began to have episodes of tachycardia during her second pregnancy, when she was 29. 'At any time of day or night my heart would speed up. During giving birth it went so fast that I lost consciousness.' The doctors thought this was due to the stress of an 'older' pregnancy and to the fact that Zoë had a very large baby (10 lb 10 oz). Zoë's heart began to speed up once again on a regular basis when she was in her early forties, causing her anxiety and increased exhaustion after each episode.

I was given beta blockers which didn't really help. I also went to a homoeopathic practitioner who indicated that my heart rate was due to a stressful life and job and the wrong diet. I then ate fewer dairy products, but it didn't make any difference. What was sometimes helpful was the use of breathing and pressure to control the fast rate once it had started. It was only when I began to have very severe and regular episodes, some lasting several hours, especially at night, and repeated visits to the local accident and emergency services, that full investigations began.

Zoë suffered over three years of these frightening episodes before she underwent radio-frequency ablation at Papworth Hospital. While waiting for a date for the operation she had to stop work for six months. She found this time depressing and lonely and she used it by beginning to communicate with her heart differently, through her imagination and visualisation.

Trying to get a feel for what was happening, Zoë had the

image of two horses in the same field. One was a young horse who wanted to break free, to run in waves in affirmation of life, to acclaim: 'I'm alive!' The other horse felt old and weary. It wanted to go into the corner of the field and give up. In pondering on the two images Zoë felt that they could well correspond with aspects of herself. She was at a mid-life point after a lifetime of responsibility and demand, almost too tired to cope with change. But she could see that she had once had the life and energy of the young horse and it was this horse who was making his presence felt now in the way this energy seemed to be dancing dangerously inside her heart. It was as if the two parts of her had become complete opposites, like the two horses in the same field. One was overburdened with responsibility, exhausted and fearing life was over; the other was still young and fresh and 'daft as a brush', as she put it. She wanted to get in touch with that energy again, but safely, and she began by allowing the very tired horse to rest and just eat grass while watching the other horse be playful. This was mirrored in her own life as she began her enforced rest from work and, when her energy allowed, to be playful by creating imaginative Christmas cards, decorations and gifts for friends. She says:

> Listen to your heart, it does 'talk'. Try to respect it, giving it time to be and yourself time to listen. Ask questions and more questions. Accept that medical knowledge is not complete or always accurate and the bottom line is that it is your heart and not someone else's. So get all the information you can, but *you* make the decisions.

Ventricular Tachycardia (VT)

These palpitations are the most serious. Here an area of the ventricle (pump) triggers a circuit or race-track movement of heartbeats within the ventricle. This makes the heart go very fast.

The Causes of VT

The most frequent cause of VT is coronary artery disease and a previous heart attack. It can also be due to cardiomyopathy (dilated, hypertrophic or arrthymogenic right ventricular dysplasia). Occasionally the condition occurs without any apparent reason.

Symptoms of VT

In short-lived – self-terminating – episodes there will be palpitations, breathlessness or chest pain. Very rapid heartbeats which last longer are often associated with near blackouts, complete blackouts or even sudden death. If you are with someone when this happens, a sharp thump to the front of the chest can sometimes stop these.

Treatment of VT

Usually electrical studies of the heart will be performed (by centres specialising in the conduction system) to assess whether tablets will stop the race-track. Sometimes ablation therapy can help, and in other cases a type of pacemaker (ICD) is implanted in the body. The pacemaker senses the abnormal rhythm and delivers a shock to the heart to stop the rhythm disturbance.

In a study of patients who were undergoing investigations of these types of rhythm disturbance, 21 per cent were found to have ventricular tachycardia in response to an emotional trigger, often surges of anger and fear.

Heart Block and Pacemakers

As already mentioned, every part of the heart has the ability to generate a heartbeat. Normally this is about 70 beats per minute, but when the heartbeat starts from the ventricle (pump), because the conducting tissue above it has been damaged by disease, the resulting heart rate is about 30 to 35 beats per minute. When this occurs it is called heart block. This can make you feel extremely weak and generally unwell.

To bring your heart back to about 70 beats a minute, a permanent pacemaker will need to be inserted. Putting a pacemaker in is quite straightforward and is done under local anaesthetic, sometimes with some sedation. The operation is performed by a cardiologist. It usually only takes between half an hour to an hour and you will only be kept in hospital for two to three days. A lead is passed into the heart from a vein near the shoulder or under the collar-bone and placed in the right ventricle. It has little attachments to the end of it so that it beds down in the heart. Sometimes a second lead is passed into the right atrium (receiving chamber), so that the top and bottom part of the heart can work better. The pacemaker battery is about the size of a matchbox but usually much flatter, and weighs about 2–4 oz (50–100 g). The battery is usually made of lithium and has a lifespan of about 10 years, after which it can easily be replaced. The battery is connected to the leads, and electrical impulses from the battery are sent down the leads to make the heart contract. The battery is inserted in a pocket under the skin near the collar-bone, and is often very unobtrusive.

If there is only one lead the heartbeat is set to a fixed rate of about 70 beats per minute; sometimes single leads can sense a requirement for an increased heart rate by vibration or changes in temperature. More sophisticated pacemakers make the heart beat only when the person's heart misses a beat (demand pacemakers). Using two leads is an attempt to make the heart beat in a more normal fashion, with the atria starting the heartbeat and the ventricles following. There are also some specialised pacemakers that recognise fast heart rates and interrupt them, so stopping blackouts. It is possible to 'question' the pacemaker battery and find out all about it and even programme it through the skin after it has been inserted, so changes can be made without further operations, and it is possible to detect when the battery starts to fail or any other problems.

Pacemakers may also be needed after operations. In these cases the surgeon attaches the wires directly to the surface of the heart. The pacemaker battery is then inserted in a little pocket in the abdominal wall.

Initials such as DDD or VVIR are often used to describe pacemakers. The three initials represent the part(s) of the heart that are paced, the part(s) of the heart that the wire senses, the person's own heartbeat and the mode of the pacemaker. Sometimes a fourth initial indicates if the pacemaker responds to activity. An ICD is a type of pacemaker that senses when the heart goes into a very fast rhythm, such as ventricular tachycardia (VT), and then delivers a small shock (defibrillator) into the heart. The 'box' with all its smart electronics is usually placed under the skin.

JOHN MCCORMICK

John went into third-degree heart block over a period of four days while on holiday in Florida. He was unable to complete his exercise routine at first, he felt short of breath and finally he was unable to lift even a small case. He decided to consult a medical practitioner, his pulse was found to be 34 and he was taken as an emergency to the nearest hospital. He suffered tremendous fluid retention that added 16 lb to his regular weight! A permanent pacemaker was inserted and his heart rate returned to normal. Within 24 hours he had passed his extra pounds in urine and was happily walking around the hospital gardens before flying home to England.

Living with a pacemaker is surprisingly straightforward. Sometimes people experience more angina as their blood is now coursing regularly around their narrowed or damaged arteries, and some adjustment may be required. You may be advised to avoid electronic equipment in airports and the use of some mobile telephones. Some stores who use security equipment based upon radio frequency post notices asking pacemaker wearers to keep a distance.

As well as being life-saving, pacemakers tend to create a 'club' such as the zipper clubs of bypass patients. Their stories are amusing and show how adaptable we can all be if necessary. One amusing anecdote came from a workshop participant who said that her neighbour had been fitted with a pacemaker recently and every time he and his wife made love the garage doors flew open!

VALVULAR HEART PROBLEMS

My heart is cooled by drops of emptiness...
THICH NHAT HANH, *Call Me by my True Names*

YOUR HEART IS a system of chambers linked by valves. There are four 'no-return' valves in each ventricle. Any of these no-return valves may develop problems, but it is usually the mitral valve (between the left atrium or collecting chamber and the left ventricle or left pump) or the aortic valve (between the left ventricle or left pump) and the main artery to the body or aorta.

Stenosis

Narrowed valves are described as stenosed. Mitral stenosis (narrowing of the mitral valve) is usually associated with rheumatic fever, which is increasingly rare in the West. Aortic stenosis (narrowing of the aortic valve) is more often due to calcium being deposited on the valve as a result of ageing.

Usually there are three parts (or cusps) to the aortic valve, but sometimes a person is born with only two. Because there are only two cusps, there is more turbulent blood flow across the valve and calcium is deposited on the valve at an earlier age.

A narrowed valve makes the heart work harder to pump blood through and you may be tired and breathless, and have chest pain or even blackouts.

Regurgitant Valves

Leaky valves are called regurgitant or incompetent. Because a valve leaks, more blood has to be pumped through each time and your heart can become stretched. Again, you can feel tired and breathless.

Leaky valves may occur after rheumatic fever, or because part of the heart has become stretched or because of the original design of the valve. Mitral regurgitation is sometimes seen after heart attacks.

Mitral Valve Prolapse

This is a particular abnormality of the mitral valve in which there is more tissue in the valve than is necessary. This causes a particular click that can be heard on examination and there may be leaking of the valve.

This condition can range from the very mild to the more severe. Often the mild form may not change for years, if at all. It deserves special mention because in some people it may be associated with palpitations and chest pain. The chest pain often responds to reassurance and relaxation exercises.

Treatment of Valve Disease

At the outset, valve stenosis (narrowing) or regurgitation (leaking) may not be severe enough to require any treatment. Under these circumstances your doctor will see you periodically to examine your heart and probably perform an echocardiogram (an ultrasound of the heart). Ultimately, the valve will need to be replaced. The timing depends on the severity of your symptoms, the size of the ventricle and the degree of narrowing or leakage that is occurring. Sometimes ACE inhibitors are given to people with leaky valves to help protect the left ventricle.

Balloon Valvotomy

It may be possible to dilate a narrowed or stenosed valve with a balloon. With aortic stenosis this is only possible in very young people, as it causes too much leaking or regurgitation in older people, but with mitral stenosis it can sometimes be useful at any age. The pulmonary valve is the one most commonly treated by this approach.

Valve Surgery

Open-heart surgery has revolutionised the treatment of faulty valves. Two main types of valve are used as replacement valves. A tissue valve is often porcine and mimics your native valve. A metal valve is man-made and may be constructed with a ball and socket or two leaflets which are centrally hinged and swing open when blood is pumped through. A tissue valve has a lifespan of 15–20 years; a metal one should last indefinitely.

Tissue valves are often put into either the young who are still growing, are taking part in vigorous sports or who may want to have a family (*see below*), or the more elderly. A second operation on the valve will almost always be necessary eventually with this type of valve.

Metal valves are very efficient and will not wear out so you will not need another operation; but because blood can clot on them, the blood-thinning agent Warfarin needs to be taken every day.

If you are on Warfarin and become pregnant you will need to be carefully supervised by a cardiologist. There is still controversy about the best way of giving anti-coagulants during pregnancy. In the UK it is common to change to a different drug around the sixth to twelfth week of pregnancy and return to Warfarin until just before delivery (at which time it is important to have a short-acting anti-coagulant so that any bleeding complications at delivery can be speedily dealt with). The reason for switching earlier on is that there is a very low risk to the developing baby during the time the internal organs are developing. There are those who believe that the risk of changing is so great to the mother and that the risk of Warfarin to the baby is so low that it is preferable to continue Warfarin throughout. This is considered particularly true if it is your mitral valve that has been replaced. In the United States there is a trend to change from Warfarin throughout the whole pregnancy.

Antibiotics

Anyone with an abnormal heart valve or who has had valve surgery should take antibiotics before certain types of dental treatment. Everyone has bacteria in their mouth, which can be sent into the bloodstream by some dental procedures. Usually this is not a problem, but a faulty or replaced valve draws bacteria to it and can set up an infection called endocarditis. This is difficult to eradicate and needs treatment in hospital, often for several weeks. Prevention is better than cure.

Similarly, antibiotics should be taken when giving birth. Until a few years ago it was considered that they were only needed if a cut (episiotomy) or forceps delivery was required, but it is now felt that it is better to give antibiotics to all who need them as sometimes in the pressure of the moment anti-biotics may be forgotten.

There has also been a recent case reported of a young man contracting endocarditis through having a number of tattoos. So it probably makes sense to have antibiotic cover for this, too. Ear piercing usually doesn't cause a problem, but it can go septic and piercing of other body parts may also get infected. Antibiotic cover seems reasonable under these circumstances.

Congenital and Inherited Heart Conditions

The word 'congenital' means 'from birth'. When a heart abnormality has been present from birth, even if it is not recognised until later, it is called congenital heart disease.

Congenital heart disease affects about 8 babies out of every 1,000 and in about half of these the abnormality is minor and will not require treatment. In the rest an intervention is required. This may involve surgery or inserting a special tube (catheter) temporarily to open up or close down various holes in the heart. Just occasionally this may cure the problem totally. In most cases, however, it only alleviates the condition to some extent. Even so, a good quality of life is usually anticipated, although further operations may be required.

The most common abnormality is a hole between either the two receiving chambers (atria), called an atrial septal defect (ASD), or between the two pumping chambers (ventricles), called a ventricular septal defect (VSD). In other instances there may be a narrowing of a heart valve (stenosis) or a major artery (for example coarctation), some of the connecting valves (atresia) may be missing, the major arteries may be misconnected (transposition) or there may only be one pumping chamber and one receiving chamber.

The Causes of Congenital Heart Disease

The cause of heart disease in babies and children is often not known, although in some cases it appears that a gene defect can cause malformation of the baby's heart in the early stages. Usually congenital heart disease is not inherited and is not due to anything that has happened to the mother during the pregnancy, German measles (rubella) being an exception. Heart abnormalities can also be associated with conditions such as Down's syndrome, Turner's syndrome and Noonan's syndrome.

Although congenital heart disease often doesn't run in families, if you have a congenital heart condition yourself or you have already had a baby with a congenital heart problem there is an increased risk – probably of about 3 per cent (that is, around 1 in 30). The risk is rarely greater. Your doctor or a geneticist will be able to give you more specific information.

Symptoms of Congenital Heart Conditions

In some cases a problem with a baby's heart is recognised when it is still in the womb (following a foetal echocardiogram); in other cases the doctor may hear a murmur when listening to the heart after birth. Normally when listening to the heart, only the opening and closing of valves is heard – any additional noise is called a murmur. Sometimes this is caused by blood rushing energetically through a normal heart; this is called an 'innocent' or 'benign' murmur. Sometimes a murmur is first picked up at a school medical or at an examination for another reason. Occasionally congenital heart conditions are not detected until adult life.

A baby with a heart abnormality often feeds badly, grows poorly and may be blue (this is due to blood bypassing the lungs). Such babies often tire easily and do not have much energy. Sometimes the baby or child may be quite well, but surgery may be advised in childhood anyway. This is because doctors recognise that problems will develop in later life and can be avoided by operating early.

Congenital heart conditions can result in a person being 'blue', or cyanosed. This occurs when there is mixing of the red and blue blood in the heart so that less red blood, which carries oxygen, gets to the tissues. The body tries to compensate for this by producing more red blood cells so that more oxygen can be carried. This is very sensible for a time, but an overproduction (polycythaemia) can lead to headaches, tiredness and sometimes gout. To relieve these symptoms, some of the red blood cells can be taken off into the sort of bag used by blood donors. This procedure is called a venesection. Only small amounts should be taken off at any one time and an equal amount of replacement fluid should be given into another vein at the same time. This is very important and you should remind any doctor who is doing a venesection that it is vital.

Living with Congenital Heart Disease

Many children with congenital heart disease remain well. Even if they have no symptoms, however, it is important that they are checked annually. This should continue in adult life at adult congenital heart disease clinics.

People born with congenital heart disease who live to become adults have often endured many operations and hospital visits and are amazing stoics. They have often had a difficult time with schooling and not being able to take part in activities with friends. They do have special problems, which need a sympathetic ear and counselling, which the Grown Up Congenital Heart (GUCH) Association or the local specialist adult congenital heart clinic can help with (*see Resources, page 251*).

Some congenital heart conditions can lead to problems during pregnancy. Usually, if you are not blue, it will be possible to have a baby. If you are blue it may still be possible, although the baby may not grow very well due to lack of oxygen delivered by the placenta. If you are blue and have a condition where the blood pressure in the lungs is the same as that in the body (Eisenmenger's syndrome) then it is very dangerous to have a baby and you may die. Irrespective, you will usually need close supervision by a cardiologist, obstetrician and anaesthetist during the pregnancy and the delivery.

If you are very blue, you may need to have oxygen when you fly in an aircraft. You will need to phone the airline involved and arrange this in advance. Many charge for the service, but there are some that do not. At the time of printing these include KLM UK, European Aviation Charter, Monarch, Qantas, Virgin Atlantic and Virgin UK.

Inherited Familial Conditions

Inherited heart conditions are due to a genetic abnormality. Sometimes this has occurred spontaneously and there is no previous family history of the condition, but the offspring of that individual are likely to inherit the condition.

In some cases the problems associated with the condition are not apparent until adult life. Usually the heart has all the right connections and the problem is due to abnormalities of the building blocks of the circulation such as the heart muscle or the connective tissue.

Marfan's Syndrome

In 90 per cent of cases this is an inherited condition. If one parent is affected then 50 per cent of the offspring are likely to have the condition, although not always to the same degree. In 10 per cent of cases Marfan's syndrome occurs out of the blue, although increasing paternal age is a factor.

The underlying problem is due to a weakness in the connective tissue of the body. Affected individuals are usually tall with very long arms (arm span greater than height) and long fingers. They are often short-sighted and have other eye problems. Their joints are very mobile – they may be double-jointed – and sometimes there are deformities of the chest wall (pectus excavatum or pectus carinatum) and the spine (kyphosis or scoliosis).

Heart problems are present in 30–60 per cent of people with Marfan's syndrome. In 35 per cent the main artery from the heart (aorta) slowly distends (dilates) and makes the aortic valve leak (aortic regurgitation); in 38 per cent the aorta may burst (aortic dissection); in 22 per cent the mitral valve leaks (mitral regurgitation).

Regular examination of the heart, usually with the help of an ultrasound machine, allows the various abnormalities to be documented and the cardiologist to decide if and when an operation is required.

The Marfan Association (*see Resources, page 251*) offers

support and advice for people with the condition and their families.

Hypertrophic Cardiomyopathy

Hypertrophic cardiomyopathy is sometimes called HOCM. It is another condition which is often hereditary and is associated with very thick, bulky muscle of either the left ventricle (usually) or the right ventricle (rarely) or (sometimes) both. It is probably familial in at least 50 per cent of cases, and if one parent is affected there is a 50 per cent chance of the offspring having the condition. Sporadic cases do occur.

If you suffer from hypertrophic cardiomyopathy you may often feel breathless and have chest pain. You may sometimes have palpitations and blackouts. The condition may be diagnosed by a murmur being heard or the characteristic features being seen on either the electrocardiogram (ECG) or the echocardiogram ('echo'). The symptoms usually develop slowly and they do not cause a significant limitation of lifestyle, but there is a subset of individuals who may die suddenly from the condition.

Tablets such as beta blockers, verapamil or amiodarone may be helpful, and sometimes an operation to trim back some of the thickened muscle is performed. Special pacemakers may also be inserted.

See page 251, Resources section for details of the patients' association – the Hypertrophic Cardiomyopathy Association.

Chapter **8**

CARDIAC TESTS AND MONITORING

A feeling heart is a blessing that no one, who has it,
would be without...
SAMUEL RICHARDSON

THERE ARE MANY tests that can be carried out to determine the condition of the heart. Some of these are routine, non-invasive procedures, while others involve passing wires or catheters into the body and are performed under local or general anaesthetic (invasive).

Non-invasive Testing

Blood Testing

If you are admitted to hospital with a heart attack, you will be given blood tests on three days. These are used to measure the levels of enzymes called CPK and LDH, which are released into the blood after there has been damage to the heart muscle (infarction).

If you are admitted with recent chest pain or unstable angina, you will undergo a blood test to measure the Troponin T or I level. Again, this measures muscle damage within the last 24 hours. It is very quick and if it is positive you will be kept in hospital; if it is negative it means that it is unlikely that serious injury to the heart has occurred.

Other routine blood tests look for the amount of haemoglobin in the blood, which is important for carrying oxygen to the tissues. If this is low, as it can be with anaemia, then it may provoke angina more quickly. The level of electrolytes (sodium, potassium, urea and creatinine) shows how the kidneys are functioning and liver function tests report on that organ's activity. Often, blood may be taken to look for overactive or underactive thyroid (thyroid function tests).

Cholesterol testing is also important and the first time this is done a fasting sample – when blood is taken first thing in the morning when you have not eaten for 12 hours beforehand – will be used to measure the triglycerides in the blood.

If you are taking Warfarin your blood will be tested to check the length of time it takes to clot against a standard known as the international normalised ratio, or INR. This will then be expressed as a ratio, for example 2.5 times longer than the standard ratio of 1. The Warfarin booklet is then updated. (This is a booklet you are given when you are started on Warfarin, in which each of the INR results is written, together with your current dose of Warfarin.) Often a target range is indicated, such as 2.5 to 3 for people with atrial fibrillation and 3 to 4 for people with valve replacements. A high figure (for example 7 or 8) indicates that the blood is too thin and there is an increased chance of bleeding complications. The Warfarin will be stopped and occasionally it may be necessary to reverse its effect with vitamin K injections. A low figure (less than 2) means that the blood is not thin enough and the Warfarin dosage will need to be increased.

ECG Tests

In an ECG test electrodes are put on your four limbs and from this a simple picture of the heart's rhythm is obtained (this is helpful if looking for irregular heartbeats such as atrial fibrillation). Electrodes are also placed across the chest wall in six places. If you are a man parts of the chest may need to be shaved. With the information from all these leads it is possible to show areas of damage (infarction), ischaemia (angina) or thickening (hypertrophy).

Exercise Tests

The electrodes are applied as above. The target heart rate is calculated by taking your age from a standard figure (220). The aim of the exercise test is to reach the age-expected target heart rate without problem – for example, if you are 50 years old you should be able to exercise to a heart rate of 170 (220 minus 50) beats per minute without symptoms or ECG changes. The test is performed either on a static bicycle or on a moving platform called a treadmill. With both tests, the amount of work you are required to do is increased every three minutes until the target heart rate is reached, or stopped sooner because of symptoms or changes on the ECG. Your blood pressure is taken before, during and after the test. This also gives important information. The ECG technician will never force you to do more than you feel able to do, but the longer you can exercise for, the more information you will provide for the doctor.

There are a number of so-called protocols for exercise testing that relate to the amount of exercise done. For out-patient testing the Bruce protocol is used. This increases the work done by a standard amount every three minutes and so can be compared with similar tests done in other hospitals. After a heart attack a Naughton protocol is often used. This is not so energetic, only lasts for six minutes and is a very good guide for subsequent rehabilitation.

Holter Monitoring

Twenty-four-hour electrocardiograms are very helpful in looking for rhythm disturbances that happen often during a

day but seemingly never at the hospital or surgery. Two electrodes are attached to your chest wall and a small box – about
the size of a portable cassette machine – is strapped on a belt
around your waist. There is a small button to press if you have
your typical symptoms and a diary to note down the time. The
tape machine has a timer built in with which to correlate your
symptoms and the ECG recording.

Cardiomemo

These are small recorders like a dictaphone which you may be
given for a month or two if you only have palpitations inter-
mittently. When your symptoms occur, the recorder is placed
over your heart or against your pulse and a short ECG recording is made. This can then often be transmitted by telephone to
an ECG technician.

Ambulatory Blood Pressure Monitoring

As already mentioned (*see page 98*), this is where a blood pressure cuff is applied to your arm and inflated every 20 minutes
for 24 hours. The results are documented on a recorder
attached to your waist and then can be read on a computer to
see how your blood pressure fluctuates through the day.

This is very helpful if your blood pressure is regarded as
borderline and in assessing your response to treatment.

Echocardiography

This technique, also known as an 'echo', uses ultrasound
waves. A probe is placed on your chest wall with some sticky
gel to allow the waves to reach the heart. The waves scan the
heart so quickly that the human eye cannot keep up, so a two-
dimensional picture is produced on a screen.

The echocardiogram is useful for looking at heart muscle
function, valves and aorta. Often a noise is produced by the
Doppler part of the probe, which looks for movement of blood

within the heart. It is a very useful investigation and is completely harmless and pain-free. Occasionally, echoes are performed after a 'stressor', such as exercise or an injection of a drug, to look at the functioning of the heart muscle. This is called stress echocardiography.

Nuclear Medicine

Sometimes exercise testing alone does not give enough information about the way your heart is functioning, but it is possible to create an image of the heart by tagging some of your blood cells with a short-acting radio-isotope. When the heart is scanned, the nuclear probe picks up the distribution of these labelled cells. This is known as a MIBI scan.

A MIBI scan is typically used when assessing blood flow to the heart muscle. A resting image is taken and then the next day a second scan is taken after something has occurred that will alter the distribution of blood. This 'stressor' may be a typical exercise test or, in people who cannot exercise due to arthritis, lung disease or some other cause, the injection of a drug, such as dipyridamole, which causes dilatation of normal (but not abnormal or atheromatous) coronary arteries.

Magnetic Resonance Imaging

This form of creating an image involves the hydrogen ions in the cells of the body which, when in a magnetic field, will align themselves so that a picture can be displayed on a screen. It involves lying still for about 20 minutes in a magnetic field while the image is produced. It cannot be performed if you have a pacemaker or certain types of artificial heart valve.

This investigation is particularly useful when looking at the structure of the heart, for example in congenital heart disease or in certain types of heart muscle condition (such as sarcoid or amyloid).

CT Scanning

CT scanning using computed tomography allows slices of X-rays to be taken of your body. These scans are often used to look at the aorta from the aortic valve around to the diaphragm. They involve lying still for a short period of time under an X-ray scanner and can be performed if you have a pacemaker or artificial heart valve.

Tilt Testing

This test is done if you have been having falls. You lie on a table and your heart rate and blood pressure are taken. Then, over a period of 40–50 minutes, the angle of the table is changed so that you are lying at an angle with your head tilted up. This can sometimes show up a marked slowing of the heart rate or change in blood pressure that will need treatment.

Invasive Testing

Angiogram

An angiogram is where a catheter – a hollow tube – is inserted into an artery to investigate the function of the heart.

If you are going to have an angiogram, you will have usually attended a pre-angiogram clinic where a nurse will have checked your blood test results and the reason for the angiogram.

Angiograms are increasingly done on a day-case basis and you will often arrive for your test 'starved', that is not having eaten for six hours beforehand. Sometimes sedation is given before you go down to the cardiac catherterisation laboratory or suite for the test, and if you are nervous and want this, ask for it.

An angiogram is usually performed from the arm (brachial) or groin (femoral). If it is done from the groin, the area will be shaved beforehand. You will be placed on a movable X-ray table which is slightly hard. There will usually be a television screen on one side so that you can see the pictures of your heart if you want to. A nurse will be beside you throughout to reassure you. The doctors will 'scrub up' – wash their hands very carefully with antiseptic soap and then put on sterile gowns and gloves. Green sterile towels will be placed around your elbow or groin, and a local anaesthetic will be injected to numb the area. It will sting a little to start with. After this has been given time to work, a doctor will insert the catheter into the artery. This is connected to a pressure tracing to show the arterial pressure and advanced towards the heart.

The catheter will be placed in first the right and then the left coronary arteries. It is often necessary to change the size and shape of the catheter for the different arteries and size of people. X-ray contrast fluid is then injected down the catheter and into each of the coronary arteries. Different views of each artery are taken with the 'arm' of the X-ray machine moving around to view the artery from other perspectives. Injection into the arteries may occasionally result in a little angina, and you may need to have a puff of GTN. Sometimes you may be asked to cough after an injection to speed the heart rate up a little.

A different catheter is usually inserted into the left ventricle and a larger amount of X-ray contrast fluid is injected using an injection pump. This will give you a short-lived hot flush. It is sometimes necessary to repeat the injection pump X-ray contrast in the aorta to look for enlargement of the aorta or leaking of the aortic valve.

Sometimes catheters are inserted into a vein (from the arm or the leg) to look at the right side of the heart and the lungs (this is called a right heart catheter), and measurements of pressure and samples of oxygen concentration are taken. Sometimes X-ray contrast fluid is injected into the right ventricle or pulmonary artery.

If the procedure has been undertaken from the groin, either the doctor or a nurse will press on the area, or a specially devised clamp will be used to stop bleeding from the site. This usually takes 15 minutes. There may be a bruise and it will feel a bit sore.

If the procedure has been undertaken from the arm, the hole in the artery will be stitched up. The stitches will need to be removed seven days later. If you are discharged that day, someone should drive you home and you should have a quiet night.

Electrophysiological Study (EPS)

This investigation into the heart's conducting system is usually undertaken from the groin. The preparation, sedation and local anaesthetic are as for the angiogram (*see above*). A number of wires (up to six) are inserted through the femoral vein and advanced to different parts of the right atrium and ventricle, and measurements are made of electrical timings.

Sometimes during the test the heart is speeded up intentionally by pacing to see if this will trigger a rhythm disturbance. As this is a controlled setting these are always corrected. On other occasions a drug may be used to see if it prevents an arrhythmia occurring.

Transoesophageal Echocardiography (TOE)

A transoesophageal echocardiogram is a test that allows a doctor to look at your heart very closely – but from the back of the heart. Your digestive tract (oesophagus) lies directly behind your heart and by passing a probe into this tract your heart can be seen very well. The tip of the probe is passed into your mouth and then advanced into the oesophagus. The probe is a long, flexible tube (about the size of your finger) which contains a special machine at the tip (transducer) to allow pictures of the heart to be sent back.

You will not be allowed to eat or drink anything for six hours before the test. Usually an anaesthetic will be sprayed on to the back of your throat, and often you will be injected with a short-acting sedative to make you feel sleepy and relaxed. This is reversed at the end of the procedure. To keep your mouth open and to protect the probe, a plastic mouthpiece will be placed gently between your teeth.

When the doctor passes the probe into your oesophagus it will not cause you any pain, nor will it interfere with your breathing at any time. It takes up to 15 minutes to examine all areas carefully. If you get a lot of saliva in your mouth during the test, the nurse will clear it using a sucker. Once the examination is finished the tube will be removed easily and quickly.

After the test you will have to wait for about an hour before you can have a drink – that is because the back of the throat has been numbed and this needs time to wear off, just like at the dentist. The back of your throat may feel sore for the rest of the day. You will need someone to drive you home and you should rest quietly for the remainder of the day, as the sedation lasts longer than you think. The effects of the test and the injection should have worn off by the next day and you should be able to resume normal activities.

Self-help

Make sure that you know what any test is for, why you need it and what it will involve. In an emergency you may not be able to do this, but later, when the crisis has passed, you will need to know what has happened to you.

Some testing, such as the treadmill test and the coronary angiogram, is helped by your own attitude and participation. In treadmill testing it is important that you are in control of the process, not the victim of someone else speeding up the floor beneath your feet. You can ask to be consulted when speed is to be accelerated, so that you can gear yourself up for more effort. You may be helped by wearing earphones playing your favourite music, something to encourage you and spur you on.

NORMAN

Norman Cousins, the man who 'laughed himself back to health', as recorded in *Anatomy of an Illness*, writes about his two very different exercise test experiences in *The Healing Heart*. His first test was associated with fear because of associations with friends who had suffered and because it was in the early days following his heart attack. He felt overwhelmed by the test and it was stopped quickly. The test results indicated to the doctors in charge that Cousins needed bypass surgery during the next week.

But Cousins knew about the power of emotional stress, such as fear and anxiety. He asked for time, and in that time prepared himself psychologically to take charge of his body. He read a great deal about the current research into heart disease and in particular the research findings on coronary artery plaque build-up and coronary spasm.

Six months later he agreed to take a further test. He had prepared himself to calm his fear by choosing different kinds of audio tapes – a Woody Allen cassette to offset the grim atmosphere of the treadmill test room and some Bach and Beethoven recordings. He asked to be in charge of the mechanism that raises the speed of the incline movement. He practised his breathing according to the output his body was demanding. In the second test he was able to continue exercising beyond the recommended time and his heart rate and blood pressure were satisfactory. He was neither breathless nor in pain. The surgery did not go ahead at that time. A year later he underwent successful bypass surgery.

In coronary angiography it is helpful to begin relaxation exercises some time before the investigation. You may be offered Valium to help you relax. This does help, as does your own breathing, relaxation or self-hypnosis technique. Visualisation can also be very supportive. Imagining yourself in a beautiful place surrounded by a wonderful landscape, and bringing in the sounds and fragrances of that place, can be very helpful in transporting you from the intensity of the procedure. Medical staff are there to reassure you and to hold your hand if you would like this and some staff do have music playing. But this is *your* body and *your* time, and you can decide what you need as support. John actually went to sleep during his angiogram; he was so laid back and good at putting himself elsewhere! Imagining your blood vessels as relaxed and wide open to accommodate the catheter is also helpful.

PART THREE

The Female Heart and the Male Heart

Chapter 9

THE GENDER OF THE HEART

A merry heart doth good like a medicine.

PROVERBS 17:22

IT IS INTERESTING to ponder on the gender of the heart – what might it be? In French, heart – *coeur* – is given the masculine gender and associated with courage and passion. Other expressions of the heart tend to favour a more feminine language and be associated with feeling and love – 'My love is like a red, red rose.'

Your actual heart is gender-free of course and there is no appreciable difference in size between a male and female heart. The differences begin in relation to body size and the way in which we use the heart – physiologically from our genetic predisposition and hormones, and psychologically through our consciousness. At times we may feel that our heart has masculine qualities such as focus, physical strength and courage; at other times feminine qualities such as receptivity, feeling and intuition. And yet all these qualities, though they are designated either 'masculine' or 'feminine', can be expressed whether you are a man or a woman.

These matters can be difficult and contentious, but it is helpful to consider how we use the vehicle of the heart or expect the heart to nurture and support us. Are we using or expecting masculine or feminine qualities? What might this tell us about our heart? Listening to your language, particularly the words you use to motivate, drive, take care of and support yourself in your everyday life, is part of the dialogue you may develop with your heart.

If, for example, you are a woman and use your heart as if you were a man, with masculine attitudes dominant, is it that you have rejected or repressed your own femininity? Or that you think masculine qualities are superior? A man may force the softer aspects of his heart to fit in with masculine stereotypes of the successful fighter, may reject his masculine consciousness in favour of something 'softer' or even give his heart over to a woman to take care of. Either way, women and men are not utilising their masculine and feminine potential.

C. G. Jung was the first psychologist to label the energies in people with masculine or feminine qualities, and archetypal structures he named anima and animus. He drew upon nature, upon ancient mythologies and deities that seemed to carry these two energies very powerfully. He named the energies of anima as being connected to the feminine, the goddesses, the energy of yin, having a soulful, diffuse, earth and water quality, and being behind procreation, the deepening of event into experience, the capacity for relatedness and forms of feminine feeling. Animus, connected to masculine yang energy and the gods, was more focused and directional, with an air and fire quality, the capacity for discipline, order and creation, and masculine rather than feminine feeling.

Jungian analysts such as Andrew Samuels and Ann Shearer have amplified an understanding of these two extremely important poles of expression to include both sexes having anima and animus as archetypal energies, ready to ignite both masculine and feminine aspects of consciousness. Qualities such as deep intuition, feeling and wisdom seem to occur when both masculine and feminine dance together.

When masculine and feminine are seen as absolutes they become polarised. So do other 'opposites'. This causes great tension between them. Things are either black or white, right or wrong. We love or hate. We suffer and want to blame others for that suffering. When we focus our attention at one end of the polarity we fear the other – when we strive to be 'good', for example, we fear the bad as very bad indeed, instead of being able to embrace both good and bad as 'good enough'. All this creates limitation and emotional stress.

When we can embrace both masculine and feminine qualities in ourselves and in other people, there can be a union of opposites and an emergence of something that goes beyond the limitations posed by absolutes. This can bring us closer to the quality of compassion and compassion is needed for healing. When we can be compassionate with ourselves, with our own thoughts, feelings, failures, losses, sadnesses and disappointments, we soften our attitude. We prevent the hardening down into absolutes that creates division and polarisation. *And in so doing, we soften and open our heart rather than hardening it against the world.*

CYRIL

An example of the effect of working with opposites came during work with a patient who came into psychotherapy because of depression and severe pains in his chest that had been hard to diagnose.

During the sessions Cyril expressed his 'heartache'. He felt a great bitterness after retirement, that he had nothing left. We discovered that he had divided his inner world into two areas: the rosy glow of the past, which was wonderful but no longer there and which seemed to carry his masculine identity, and the grey misery of the present and future, which seemed to symbolise a weak femininity, fuelling his bitterness. In putting down his current life because he judged it by the past expectations, he was wiping out his entire life experience on a daily basis and was also unable to live in the present moment or enjoy any of his creative capacity.

In realising this, and in monitoring how often his thinking about his world and choices was dominated by this polarity, he began to be able to *be* with his present experience and reclaim many facets of himself that he had rejected. He started walking in the woods near his home and began to create artwork again.

The culmination of his work with these extreme polarities was a dream in which he pulled a beautiful ancient sculpture of a man's head out of a flowing river. He felt that the river indicated that his attitude to feeling and his inner life were moving again and that his connection with them had brought him a gift. He was able simply to be sad instead of bitter, and he began to be more present in the moment. He continued making things out of clay and wood, something he had not done for 20 years, without judging them. He became kinder to his body. The tightness in his body, his shallow breathing, the severity of his chest pain and his depression were dissolved through this process of shifting energy and attitude.

The Masculine and Feminine in You

Spend a few moments just thinking about what you consider masculine and feminine. Make two columns and write down the words and images you regularly use to refer to masculine and feminine. You might have masculine and feminine role models, people who have inspired you or people who carry stereotypes you dislike. Joan of Arc, Joan Collins, Margaret Thatcher, Posh Spice, Mother Teresa and Princess Diana are some female figures who may offer a 'hook' for your feminine projections. William the Conqueror, Bill Clinton, Darth Vader, David Beckham, St Francis of Assisi and the Dalai Lama might offer a hook for masculine projections. Try and stay with descriptive qualities and feelings rather than roles.

Then monitor (by writing in a notebook) how often you think in an 'if ... then' or an 'either ... or' way about yourself, your choices and your life, for example: 'If I'm not a conquering hero like Boadicea or Alexander the Great, then I'm a hopeless wimp.' The consequences of this polarised thinking is that if we 'fail' to be like Boadicea or Alexander the Great we presume we are a wimp and give up on ourselves. Here is another one: 'If I'm kind, soft and accepting, then I will be taken advantage of, even abused.' Here we might be hardening our heart because of a 'false' premise that became rooted in our thinking years ago and is in need of revision.

Here are some more examples of opposites to add to those we can divide into masculine and feminine, taken from the 'dilemmas' in the psychotherapy file used in Cognitive Analytic Therapy at Guy's and St Thomas's hospitals:

'If ... then' or 'Either ... or'

◆ 'I feel as if I have no choice but to be either busy career person or carer, or lonely and alone.'

◆ 'If I am successful I feel guilty, as if I have to pay a price for success, so I play down my achievements or don't try at all.'

◆ 'I tend to bottle up my true feelings for fear of becoming over-emotional.'

◆ 'I repress and store angry feelings, feeling a martyr while others are brutes.'

◆ 'I strive for perfect control because I am afraid of perfect mess.'

◆ 'I tend to placate others and then find myself bingeing out of unmet need.'

Monitor this polarised thinking for about a week. See what this brings forth and where these dilemmas are rooted in your past. You can revise them by asking: 'Does this need to be so now?' Then see if you can soften these extremes within your-self in order for a third position to emerge.

The Super-achieving Man and Woman

In 1974 Meyer Friedman and Ray Rosenmann were the first doctors to study the behaviour and personalities of people with heart disease. They found that a certain type of personality, which they called 'Type A personality', was at much greater risk of heart disease than the so-called 'Type B personality'. Their later studies, which looked for the developmental cause of the Type A personality, began a process of building the bridge between psychology and the heart.

Friedman and Rosenmann's studies have inspired other work on how emotional behaviour affects the heart. More importantly, specifying risk behaviour and its original roots has helped health professionals not just to look for these types, but actively to work with the behaviour within them once identified. Now other cardiologists and doctors working with heart patients, Dr Dean Ornish in particular, have developed holistic programmes of rehabilitation for the 'coronary-prone personality' that address wounds to the inner person and the soul as well as those to the physical heart.

Historically the coronary-prone personality described below has been attributed more to men than women, although this may be changing as more women join a competitive market-place as a means of finding personal significance.

Coronary-prone individuals frequently have an over-commitment to work, to performance and achievement, and are driven to perfection in order to produce a 'successful' self-image to the outside world. Accompanying this is a sense of urgency and impatience and free-floating hostility (anger) that can be triggered by someone or something getting in the way of the projected ideal. Even when success is accomplished in the outside world there is little personal satisfaction or fulfilment. The drive to maintain the successful self-image continues, like a relentless treadmill. This need to push yourself beyond reasonable limits of endurance has proved to be very bad for the heart.

The coronary-prone individual tends to repress spontaneity or self-expression and feels the need to control their environment. It is difficult for them to relax or accept genuine feelings of love and care. Rehabilitation programmes, counselling or psychotherapy, or any suggestions from professionals that demand self-reflection or effort on their own behalf can inflame rage and therefore tend to be avoided. Underlying this drive to perfection and control is an enormous feeling of panic, rage at the fear involved in the panic, fear of anyone finding out and terror of weakness.

The heart of the coronary-prone individual may be defended physically by an enlarged, over-muscled chest and a posture of being 'big and brave', with the shoulders back and the chest pressed forwards in military fashion. 'Nobody gets to me' is the message from the armoured body. The eyes may reveal something quite different.

Research shows that underneath this formidable drive and probably outward success is an extremely vulnerable individual with tender and needy feelings which have never been able to find a safe outlet. It may be that in childhood love was conditional upon performance or upon being seen as 'good'. This sort of experience has different repercussions on men and women biologically and socially.

Chapter 10

THE HEART IN A WOMAN'S BODY

A pity beyond all telling is hid in the heart of love.
W. B. YEATS, *The Pity of Love*

HEART DISEASE IS often thought of as a predominantly male disease. However, it is the single greatest cause of death in women.

Every year in the UK, five times as many women die from coronary heart disease as from breast cancer. This risk increases to six times in black women. This is one of the highest death rates from heart disease in the world. Many women say that they fear breast cancer more than any other disease, yet in reality it is heart disease which is more predominant. Scottish women are especially at risk – a woman aged between 35 and 74 in Scotland has 109 times the risk of dying from heart disease than a woman in Japan. Southeast Asian women have a 50 per cent higher risk than all other UK women. A lot of research is being carried out into these statistics, but generally speaking the variations are down to ethnic origin, diet and lifestyle.

Coronary artery disease tends to occur, on average, 10 years later in women than in men because of the protective effect of female hormones up to the time of the menopause, or 'the change'. It can, however, occur in pre-menopausal women. It accounts for 25 per cent of all deaths from angina/heart attacks in those under the age of 65.

A Woman's Lifestyle

Despite the huge recent change in terms of male and female 'roles' in relationships, women are still predominately the main carers of partners, children and the elderly, and they outnumber men in the caring professions. While caring is satisfying and nourishing, too much serving of others and neglecting your own needs can be harmful. Women who have become accustomed to serving their male or female partner may become anxiously involved in looking after their loved one's heart and neglect their own. Women may criticise their partner's unhealthy lifestyle (smoking, fatty foods, lack of exercise, and so on) and not heed their own advice! Half of all adult women are overweight and 17 per cent of these are obese. Also, 28 per cent of adult women smoke and a huge 69 per cent don't exercise at all. Many women are so unfit that a normal walking pace can make them breathless.

Certain job conditions and family responsibilities are a particular source of stress in women. Working mothers in low-paid and low-status jobs have been found to have a much higher risk of heart disease than others. Depression and panic disorders also occur more often in women. Both of these are now accepted risk factors for heart disease. The changing expectations of women can lead to frustration and despair. Many women have more responsibilities than ever before – by trying to be everything to everyone they push themselves to excel in all roles, often at a cost to their physical and mental health. Women have consistently higher rates of physical and mental unwellness (morbidity) than men.

● LIFESTYLE ANALYSIS

Make a chart for yourself for each day of the last week. Colour in how much of your day was spent at work. Choose another colour for activities connected with children (collecting from school, homework, and so on), another for the chores you do for other people (shopping, cooking, laundry, and so on) and a further colour for time for yourself (time spent reading, listening to the radio, on hobbies such as sewing or painting, time spent talking and laughing with friends).

Spend a few minutes pondering on the feeling of last week. What was the highlight of your week? What nourished you most?

1. Write down what qualities you feel are demanded of you at work. Does your job come easily to you? Does it suit your temperament? Does it satisfy you? If not, what effect does it have upon you, having to produce the qualities you've written above?

2. What food did you buy and who was it for? When you prepare food, do you sit down to eat it? Is it shared with others or do you eat alone? How often do you 'eat on the run' – in the car, on the bus, while standing in a corridor waiting?

3. How often do you get time alone to do what you really want to do? If this is minuscule, or non-existent, what can you do to change this?

4. How often do you say 'no' when someone asks you to do something and you don't want to?

5. Visualise your heart. What does it look like? How is it affected by living inside your body, a woman's body? Do you imagine it would have a different life if it lived inside a man's body? Notice your reactions to this question, they might be very telling. If so, what are they telling you?

Achievement Guilt and Happiness

Women are thought to carry more guilt than men, especially women who juggle many roles as multiple carer, breadwinner, cook, bottle washer and high achiever. This may be because women have only recently been free to take their places in the job market and their consciousness has not yet adjusted. Many working mothers have said to me, 'If I don't go to work I feel guilty at just staying at home with my child, as if I've sold out after all that women have fought for, and if I go out to work I feel guilty for leaving my child with a child minder. I cannot win.'

Women often expect their bodies to do the same tasks as men and take the same strains without cost. Also, there is huge societal pressure to be a high-earning boss, fashion plate *and* kitchen goddess.

● ASSESSING THE GUILT HABIT

- Keep a notebook for one week and write down every time you feel guilty. Make a note of the time, place and what you feel guilty about. It might be that you've got angry with someone, you've only half-finished something, you haven't called your mother, you've forgotten to take something out of the freezer or you've not mended the hem of your skirt.

- Now write down each time you feel happy, joyous, content. Write down where you are at these moments, who (if anyone) is around you and what you are doing.

This exercise aims to build information about your attitude and to ascertain the compromises that you make between different roles. The aim is to embrace all aspects of your life as having a valid part to play. And if your heart needs you to take notice and to take care of yourself in a new and more intimate way, then this adjustment needs to be made as soon and as smoothly as possible.

Physical Problems – Women at a Disadvantage

Many healthcare teams still seem to be directing coronary heart disease screening clinics at men, perpetuating the myth that heart disease is mainly for men and that the risk for women is small. Continuing this misunderstanding, women still tend to minimise their symptoms because they believe that they are not at risk of heart disease (the so-called Yentl syndrome). Doctors may also not take a woman's symptoms seriously. Women with chest pain often have to wait longer than men to be seen by a specialist and are less likely to be referred for coronary angiography or bypass surgery or balloon dilatation of the arteries (angioplasty). After a heart attack men are seven times more likely to have angioplasty or surgery than women and twice as likely if they have angina. Women also appear to be less likely to have clot-busting (thrombolytic) drugs given at the time of a heart attack and are, as a result, less likely to survive the first heart attack.

Studies show that women are less likely than men to enrol in cardiac rehabilitation programmes and have a higher dropout rate. This is particularly relevant to older women (over 70) who would really benefit from such programmes. Around three to four weeks after a heart attack, women have reported increasing their activity by adding more types of household jobs, whereas men engaged in walking programmes.

Women are also more likely than men to experience depression and anxiety after a heart attack and have feelings of guilt at their inability to perform usual household activities. This has been found to be a very high source of stress in women following heart attacks. Whereas men often report family members waiting on them after a heart attack, women resist being helped with typical household chores such as meal preparation or house cleaning. There has been a great deal of research showing that women recovering from a heart attack report more life changes and increased marital and social difficulties than men.

Patterns of Chest Pain in Women

A big problem for doctors when investigating chest pain in women is that it is often not typical of heart disease and may not represent heart disease. This is called atypical or non-cardiac chest pain.

To confuse the issue further there is a subgroup of women who test positive for heart disease on an exercise test but are then found to have normal coronary arteries. This condition is called Syndrome X. Little is known about it, except that it may be associated with alterations in the tone of the smooth muscle surrounding the smaller arteries in the heart and may respond to certain types of medication such as calcium channel blockers. The women who have been told that they have heart disease and are then found to have normal coronary arteries actually need help coming to terms with this and dealing with the other possible causes of their chest pain, which include hyperventilation, phobic anxiety and depression. Confusingly, these other causes are now known to be risk factors for subsequent heart disease.

There are other causes of atypical chest pain, including mitral valve prolapse, microvascular angina (Syndrome X) and coronary artery spasm (which are given various names such as Prinzmetal, vasospastic or variant angina).

The typical chest pain in women also has some differences from that of men in that it occurs more frequently during rest, sleep or periods of mental stress. Women are also more likely to suffer from neck and shoulder pain, nausea, vomiting, fatigue and breathlessness in addition to chest pain. Since the standard exercise test with monitoring of the electrocardiogram (the ECG or electrical heart trace) may not identify heart disease properly in women or as well as it does in men, there is an increasing trend towards performing exercise and then studying the heart with either ultrasound (stress echocardiography) or with a nuclear medicine scan (MIBI scan) (*see pages 123–30*). Women's symptoms may also be less clear-cut during a heart attack, so women tend to arrive later than men at coronary care units.

High Blood Pressure and Women

Although men have a slightly greater chance of having high blood pressure, more women than men have high blood pressure after the age of 50. This reflects a number of facts:

♦ Blood pressure rises progressively with age and, on average, women tend to live longer than men. This rise with age is much greater in black women than white women, though the reasons for this are unclear.

♦ Fewer women have high blood pressure before the menopause, possibly because of higher levels of oestrogen and lower levels of male hormones (androgens) and possibly because periods reduce the amount of blood in the body in a beneficial way.

♦ High blood pressure appears to increase at a faster rate in women than men after the age of 50.

♦ An increase in body weight – which can increase blood pressure – occurs in some women after the menopause.

♦ On the positive side, women appear to have fewer complications than men with similar blood pressure levels.

FRANCES

After a diagnosis of high blood pressure, Frances made an energy map and realised her sense of isolation came from the habit of postponing arrangements to meet friends and family. She believed that if she didn't 'stay on top' of her job she would lose it, and her life with an invalid husband demanded that she stay in work. She was also proud and disliked being seen as needing help. When her husband's illness became worse, she tried to cope alone and ended up becoming unwell herself. The map helped her to restore a sense of balance and proportion in her life.

Hormone Therapies and the Heart

Many women take hormone therapies throughout their lives. Younger women who are trying to avoid pregnancy may take the contraceptive pill. Older women nearing the 'change' and its irregularity of menstrual cycles may take hormone therapy to be sure of avoiding unwanted pregnancy and stabilising many of the uncomfortable symptoms associated with the menopause. These hormones can affect the heart.

Oral Contraceptives and Coronary Risk

There is no evidence that low-dose contraceptives increase the coronary risk in women who do not smoke. Past use of oral contraceptives also does not affect coronary risk in non-smoking women. *But* high-dose oral contraceptives and smoking increase the risk seven times.

HRT and the Menopause

The average age of the onset of the menopause is 51. During the shift in body chemistry the ratio of the different parts of cholesterol are changed, lowering the protective one (HDL) and raising the harmful one (LDL). Also, the blood tends to clot more quickly because one of the levels of clotting factors (fibrinogen) increases.

Menopause may also be a time when hormonal changes associated with emotional response to stress are high. It can be a desperate, terrifying time of being enslaved by hormones, dragged down by distressing symptoms and moods. It can also be a relief, a release, a change for the better physically. The end of fertility that it brings can either be a source of regret or a huge relief. Certainly the menopause is a threshold, one which Germaine Greer describes in her excellent book *The Change* as holding the potential for a greater peacefulness and spiritual awareness than ever before. She writes:

The older woman's love is not love of herself, nor of herself mirrored in her lover's eyes, nor it is corrupted by need. It is a feeling of tenderness so still and deep and warm that it gilds every grass blade and blesses every fly. It includes the ones who have a claim on us, and a great deal besides. I wouldn't have missed it for the world.

The risks of heart disease rise as the protection of oestrogen lessens, so it is important that women learn to take care of all expressions of their heart during the onset of the menopause. In fact the passage of the menopause itself, which can last several years, can be a useful time to make subtle philosophical adjustments so that you are ready to enjoy an expressive, creative and challenging later life.

Hormone replacement therapy (HRT) is often prescribed at the menopause. The simplest form of HRT consists of oestrogen alone, but this is only suitable if you have had a hysterectomy (the womb or uterus removed). It is safer to have a combination of oestrogen and progesterone if you have not had a hysterectomy in order to protect against cancer of the uterus. This does mean that you will continue to have a withdrawal bleed. More recently it has become possible to have 'continuous combined HRT', which is more acceptable to women since it usually gives no bleeding or only light spotting in the first three to six months of use.

There is a variety of routes for HRT. These include oral pills, skin (transdermal) patches, gels and implants under the skin. HRT will also protect you from thinning of the bones (osteoporosis) and thinning of the lining of the vagina (making lubrication easier). It is said to thicken the hair and give you more energy.

There is real uncertainty about whether HRT protects against the development of coronary heart disease and whether it should be used as a preventative measure against the further development of heart disease. There are a number of major trials (including the WISDOM trial in the UK) currently ongoing which will try to answer the question as to whether HRT lowers the risk or increases the chances of developing heart attacks, breast cancer, osteoporosis and dementia.

Some recent trials have noted an increased incidence of vascular events, including heart attack, stroke and deep vein thrombosis (blood clots in the leg) in the early months of women starting HRT. The number of women actually having these events was small (less than 1 per cent) and did not meet the statistical criteria for stopping the trial – that is because it may have occurred by chance. Another study also found an increase in vascular events in the first year of HRT, followed by an apparent protective effect in later years.

The current advice is that women should certainly not stop taking HRT if it has already been prescribed, but that at the moment it should not be started if a woman has recently had a heart attack or been diagnosed with angina. If you have had a heart attack and were already taking HRT, you should continue taking it, as all the additional risks due to alteration in clotting factors which may predispose you to unstable angina have long passed.

Blood Pressure and HRT

In post-menopausal women with normal blood pressure, HRT does not raise blood pressure and may even lower it.

Fewer women develop high blood pressure after the menopause while taking HRT than would be expected.

HRT does not make the blood pressure higher in women with already high blood pressure and appears to be safe in these circumstances – in fact some studies have shown that it may even be beneficial.

The Risk of Breast Cancer

HRT can cause a twofold increase in the risk of breast cancer, but this has to be balanced by the fact that increasing age brings a dramatically increased risk of dying from heart disease as compared to breast cancer. Moreover, heart disease is considered to be the principal cause of disability in women.

The table below shows that by the time a woman has reached the age of 70 her chance of developing breast cancer during her remaining life is reduced to 1 in 29. Similarly, a woman's risk of dying of breast cancer during her remaining life decreases as her age increases. This is in contrast to her risk of dying of heart disease, which remains at an average of 1 in 3.3 throughout life.

Risk of a woman developing or dying of breast cancer or dying of heart disease during her remaining life (based on data from Office for National Statistics)

Age (years)	Risk of developing breast cancer	Risk of dying of breast cancer	Risk of dying of heart disease
30	1/12	1/24	1/3.4
40	1/12	1/25	1/3.4
50	1/14	1/26	1/3.4
60	1/18	1/30	1/3.3
70	1/29	1/37	1/3.2
80	1/57	1/48	1/3.2

So unless there is a personal history of cancer or a strong family history of breast cancer, HRT really does appear to be worthwhile, especially if you are at high risk of heart disease. You can take it even if you have high blood pressure or diabetes or have had a stroke. A recent study from Finland found that death from heart disease among 1,000 HRT users was 79 per cent lower than among women who had never used HRT.

Oestrogen Receptor Modulators

Oestrogen receptor modulators mimic the effect of oestrogen in some target tissues while blocking the effect in others. Tamoxifen (an oestrogen hormone treatment given to some women with breast cancer) is one of the earliest of these. It works against oestrogen in the breast while benefiting bone and cholesterol. It does still mimic the effect of oestrogen in the uterus and may maintain the protective effect upon the heart.

A new generation of selective oestrogen receptor modulators (SERMs) has now appeared which mimics the effect of oestrogen on bone and cholesterol and works against oestrogen in the uterus and breast, which means that there is no increased risk of uterine cancer and even a slight protective effect against breast cancer (it may reduce the risk by as much as two-thirds). It may be that this type of pill is the logical one to be on after taking HRT for 5 to 10 years. As SERMs don't reduce menopausal symptoms, they are not prescribed at the outset. Examples are Evista (Raloxifene).

Chapter 11

THE HEART IN A MAN'S BODY

My heart is a lonely hunter that hunts on a lonely hill.
FIONA MCLEOD, *The Lonely Hunter*

The Image of the Strong Man

MASCULINITY HAS TRADITIONALLY been equated with toughness, with control and success. This makes it hard for men to accept becoming ill and to express their fears and needs. Men tend to underuse medical and psychotherapeutic services and be less interested in 'self-help' for a change in either physical or emotional well-being. Taking illness 'like a man' can often mean hiding the loneliness and pain behind a brave face and weeping in private. This can cause many problems.

Head or Heart?

The idea that there is an 'either/or' – another polarity – about head or heart is still held in many men's psyches as well as in women with male psyches. The idea is that the head, or brain, is superior and the heart, or emotions, is inferior. To 'give in to' your heart is seen as weak, while 'keeping your head' at all times signifies rationality and control. This may have served well when men were the hunters, gatherers and warriors of a society. But today, away from military command or gathering food from the beast-dominated jungle, this crude survival inheritance has yet to find a new place. It is still taught, however – even at the mother's breast! Many powerful driving mothers have demanded that their sons put away 'childish' needs long before these needs had been truly met in order to be a 'proper man', or even, in worst cases, a 'better man than your father'.

'New Man' and 'Lonely Man'

Over the last few decades there has been a huge cultural change in Western societies in relation to the roles of men. While men still hold the majority of high-profile jobs, earn more money and have the loudest voices, many women are choosing to live their lives, even become mothers, without a man in sight. Many more people are getting divorced and the number of divorced mothers and fathers raising children in single-parent families is one in four. What does it do to male ego and self-esteem to be not needed for the traditional role? And what are the new roles for men in terms of families and partnerships?

A 'new man' is considered to be one who embraces tasks and attitudes previously considered female – changing nappies, carrying babies, taking time off work to look after children, making relationships a priority rather than an appendage. But does swinging in this way to the opposite pole, to heart, make 'head' more extreme as it fights for survival in the shadow? If the warrior who thrives upon testosterone is repressed, what happens to a man's natural survival aggression? All of us, men and women, need to understand and work with our own aggression, otherwise it leaks out inappropriately in revenge brutalities or in bullying, or we turn it against ourselves in addictive illnesses or depression.

To be all head and no heart is lopsided and fraught with potential emotional pain. But to reject 'head' in favour of 'heart' without being mindful of what that might mean is exactly the same. No one wishes for a masculinised woman, all brass armour and control with a sentimentalised set of emotions in her shadow; and no one wants a feminised man, all soft and floppy without focus and discipline.

The pressure of political correctness upon men to move away from the traditional male qualities such as competition, striving and winning, toughing it out, bravery, valour, honour and discipline seems a loss. Society needs these leadership qualities to be in place alongside the wisdom, relatedness and sense of timing that are considered the more feminine values. We all need a balance of head and heart, and ultimately, to be of one mind with no divisions.

Self-image

There is a tendency for men to retain a youthful self-image in their behaviour pattern. So drinking and eating habits – fatty foods, takeaways, regular hangovers – started in youth often persist into later life. Many men continue in this fashion, content that heart disease will not happen to them – or at least not yet – without realising that it can and often does strike in the twenties and thirties. A recent British Heart Foundation advertisement characterises this attitude very well.

Also, men generally tend to be overweight and not take enough exercise. Even men who have been keen sportsmen in their younger days find that as the pressures of job and family increase they no longer make time to take part in regular exercise.

Just taking the stairs rather than the lift or escalator may be enough to keep healthy. Walking to work, if feasible, or programming some time at the weekend for activity, rather than shopping or just 'vegging out', should be a priority.

A Man's Inheritance

Men carry, through their gender inheritance, one of the main risk factors for coronary heart disease – the male hormone testosterone. Heart disease in men probably has more to do with the balance of testosterone and oestrogen than with oestrogen deficiency. Protective levels of HDL (good) cholesterol are the same in boys and girls up to puberty. Women continue to have higher levels of HDL cholesterol until the menopause, when their oestrogen levels fall. HDL cholesterol starts to decline in men when testosterone levels rise at puberty. Furthermore, the number of men suffering angina and heart attacks starts to decline when they lose much of their testosterone in old age. Men may benefit from having a selective anti-androgen that balances testosterone levels.

What about Viagra?

A specifically masculine problem is that blood flow to the penis may be affected by atheroma, just like the coronary arteries. Consequently erectile dysfunction or impotence can occur. Diabetes can also cause impotence, as can drugs such as beta blockers.

Although there were some early reports linking Viagra with heart deaths, British and American expert panels have concluded that there is no causal link. Viagra prescribed by your doctor can be used if you have a heart condition as long as you are not taking long-acting forms of GTN called nitrates, or the drug Nicorandil (Ikorel), and that you do not need to use GTN before, during or after making love.

Coronary-prone Men

We have already seen that in 1974 Meyer Friedman and Ray Rosenmann were the first doctors to study the behaviour and personalities of people with heart disease. Their findings were based upon their predominately male patients, which at the time mirrored the extent to which men carried the theme of being either a super-achiever, all activity, or a man bypassed by defeat and despair. 'Coronary-prone' individuals frequently had an over-commitment to performance and achievement, coupled with impatience and free-floating hostility and difficulty in accepting genuine feelings of love and care.

For a man, since his first intimate relationship is with his mother, there may emerge an extremely ambivalent attitude towards mother, towards women, towards anything seen as 'feminine', which would include how he looks after himself and his needs. There again we have the splitting into opposites, creating the tension of polarisation. Women may be needed by the coronary-prone man externally in order to look good in the world and internally for the longed-for closeness, but the intimacy of a close relationship may threaten to reveal his unmanageable vulnerability. Because it is impossible to take a risk, or a chance in love, the rage against the restrictions imposed by receiving only conditional love may make relationships short-lived or impossible. This explains the anger towards anything vulnerable that many coronary-prone personalities, both men and women, have.

If you feel you are at risk from developing or have already developed what we are describing as the coronary-prone personality, and that these habits are your way of life, don't feel alarmed or depressed. Just the recognition itself is the first step to changing your situation. The next step is to become active on your own behalf. The different questionnaires and exercises throughout this book are designed to help you to take one step at a time towards softening and opening a redundantly armoured and hardened heart.

Isolation

Cardiologist Dean Ornish's studies on reversing heart disease and data from men's heart groups reveal men who have a store of unmet feeling and need in their heartspace. Robert Bly, pioneer of men's groups and author of the influential book *Iron John*, speaks of the huge well of feeling, in particular loss, loneliness and shame, that emerges when groups of men come together to be themselves and share rituals that allow a free flow of feeling. Much of this sense of isolation seems to have developed under the pressures of the old-fashioned approach to being 'men' and the pressure to be 'a good boy' in relation to a parent whose approval was paramount for survival.

In his book *Heartbreak and Heart Disease*, Dr Stephen T. Sinatra writes:

> As a cardiologist I see a lot of 'good boys' with heart disease. In my workshops I have learned that they carry around a lot of denial about anger – especially towards the women in their lives...

Men also carry around a lot of denial about their emotional need and need for connection. The most painful isolation is often that of being unable to connect to their own true self.

Fortunately, this is changing. Many men today are throwing away their stereotyped swords and taking up a wiser staff to climb the mountains within their own psyches as well as those within the outer world, whether in medical research, ecology, world politics or economics. The many current pioneers of research into the emotional and spiritual needs evident in heart patients are, by a huge majority, men – Deepak Chopra, Dean Ornish and Mehmet Oz, to name but a few. These male voices are crying out for both men and women to move into a much more balanced relationship with the heart in all its connotations. And this greater sense of balance is sorely needed in our current world.

Questions on Self-awareness to Reflect Upon

1. If heart disease is in your family, how has it been discussed?

> Make a family tree for yourself showing the number of men in your family with heart disease, their work, habits, age, and so on.
>
> What can you learn from this, what might be helpful? For example, if you carry the burden of genetic inheritance, how might you support yourself? By discussion,

by joining a support group, by gaining as much information about what helps to keep your heart healthy...?

2. What does it mean to you to be in a male body today?

If you were to observe your familiar body posture, how would you describe it? 'Relaxed', 'flexible', 'big and brave', 'armoured in defence', 'ready to pounce', 'always looking over your shoulder'? What do you feel is the cost of holding this position in terms of energy?

What qualities do you consider masculine?

How do you express these qualities yourself, in your life?

Who are your role models for behaviour and for work?

Do you allow yourself to express feeling? If not, what do you feel happens to your feelings? Would you like to develop more of an emotional literacy around feeling?

How might you address this, for example by being proactive on your own behalf, through reading, discussion, joining a group of like-minded men?

3. Do you allow yourself your full ambition? Try writing down what you would really like to do with your life.

4. What is your pattern in friendships and intimate relationships?

How many close male friends do you have with whom you can talk intimately about things that are really important to you, without having to be competitive or fearing vulnerability?

If you find you have few friends and tend to shy away from making the effort at contact with others you may have low self-esteem following a loss at work or in a relationship or a bereavement. It is important for your health as a whole person to do all you can to restore your confidence. You may find it helpful to speak to a counsellor or take up an activity that puts you in touch with others.

If you have a pattern of difficult, painful relationships,

would you consider psychological counselling or psychotherapy to help you understand your part in relationship patterns?

5. Men are reported to think about sex every seven minutes.

   Does this apply to you?
   How would you describe your sexual drive?
   Does this get satisfied?
   How do you cope if not?
   Do you accept sex without a relationship?

6. What hobbies or other creative pursuits nourish you? Write them down and how often you practise them.

7. What, if any, are your spiritual beliefs and practices? Have you ever considered the power of prayer, meditation or healing?

WILLIAM (*See also page 18*)

William's problems began in 1972 when, at 38, he started to get angina at rest. After eight weeks in hospital it was hoped that he might recover through the process of natural revascularisation (the healthy blood vessels in the heart taking on more work). (Smaller blood vessels, or collaterals, can be used to get around a blockage in a process called collateralisation. It may be helped by exercise and can occur at any age. Most people will develop some collaterals with time, but it is not possible to predict how much benefit will be derived.) But this didn't happen. William had one of the earliest bypass operations, in 1975. He said:

I thought when I first had angina that the problem was doing too much. I was the kind of person who didn't say 'no' if I was asked to do something. I was a university teacher, administrator, counsellor and magistrate. But in my heart I really knew that the problem was my marriage. I was told I had coronary artery disease and to wait and see.

William was advised to simplify his life and to focus on the essentials. But his job and marriage continued to be extremely demanding. During 1985 his father died, and he moved to London and had a heart attack. The period of rest in hospital gave him the permission he needed to stop, and psychotherapy helped him to have a safe place to look at the difficulties within his marriage.

> Everything that had been repressed and buried came flooding out in hospital. It was like a dam breaking and I couldn't stop talking.

Soon after this time William ended his marriage and spent several years living on his own. During this time he faced loneliness and depression while he continued looking into the patterns that had underpinned his attitudes towards life and himself. He met his second wife, with whom he now has two children, and began a happier and very different kind of life.

> What I've learned is that I cannot cope with prolonged stress without hurting myself. I have to respond to my body protesting. It's taken some time for this to sink in, and for me to respond rather than keep going stoically. What I'd like to pass on to others is that long-term disease needs long-term care. Your life may have to change quite radically in order to enhance its quality. I would say to anyone with a heart problem, 'You must work out how best to look after your arteries and yourself. It's essential that you do, and that *you never let up on this.*'

PART FOUR

Recovery and Rehabilitation

Chapter 12

RECOVERY FROM HEART ATTACK AND ANGINA

He behaved as if he could run past death itself.
WIFE OF HEART ATTACK PATIENT

AFTER THE DISCOVERY by Harvey of the circulation of the blood, the more poetic images of the heart retreated from medicine in favour of the image of the heart as a mere pump. What also retreated was the slow, contemplative approach to the care and recuperation of the heart favoured by Victorian physicians, which mainly focused on the values of rest and sleep together with the balance of rest and effort. Today, cardiology relies upon medications and interventions such as surgery, and in rehabilitation emphasis tends to be towards exercise and diet. Although less attention is given to the balance between rest and effort, rehabilitation programmes are now beginning to give more attention to this area and to psychological issues.

If you have had a heart 'event' such as a heart attack, heart operation or other heart-related problem, you will be feeling shocked. Shock affects body, mind, feelings and spirit. It takes time for it to leave your system. When we are shocked it takes more energy and thus more time to do everyday things. Give yourself the time you need. You will need to pay great attention to the small steps in everyday life and be careful not to become overstressed as you embark upon your recovery. Also, it is important not to think of heart medication or operations as a 'magic bullet' that will propel you back into life as it was before. Heart events change lives. They make us want to rethink priorities. Many people think of them as a warning and use the time offered after the warning to settle old issues and make new plans.

Heart Attack

A heart attack is always a crisis, whether you are at home or in hospital. But it need not be fatal. Statistics show that in Britain the death rate from heart attacks is between 6 and 20 per cent. The higher death rate is in those over 75 and diabetics.

Following the news that you have had a heart attack you may feel:

♦ Shocked and numb.

♦ Afraid of dying.

♦ Anxious and helpless.

♦ Frightened that you may have another attack.

♦ Worried about the implications for your health.

♦ Concerned that your activity will be limited.

♦ Overwhelmed by the new information you have to digest and decisions you have to take.

♦ Possibly ambivalent about your survival.

These are all normal feelings and have been expressed by countless heart attack patients. It is much better to name the feelings, however irrational they may seem to you, and try and speak about them to someone you trust, to get reassurance and support.

The time immediately following a heart attack is needed for

rest, so it is important to leave any other thinking or decision-making until you have more energy. Everything *has* to wait while your heart restores its equilibrium.

You may find that much talking is needed following a heart attack, for this event has implications for the whole family and may be the trigger point for many hidden feelings rushing to the surface. You will be relieved that you have survived, but may also feel angry, guilty or resentful.

Surviving a heart attack gives everyone a sharp reminder that their time is limited. Many people feel they have had a lucky escape and they move on to grasp the gift of life in a more full-hearted way, vowing to give up their bad habits and spend more time with friends and family. For those who have chosen a more solitary life, being unwell challenges them to either ask for help or organise care. Some who prefer a solitary life take themselves off to a hotel or convalescent home if they can afford it, or organise a stay with friends. For those who feel lonely, this may become more accentuated and there may be an acute sense of time running out. Sometimes there is a sense of 'weakness', or what John referred to as the 'wounded animal' who would get picked off by other animals out there in the competitive jungle of commercial life.

Learning to value 'borrowed time' takes many adjustments.

Recovery in Hospital

Hospitals are busy places and cardiac units are fine-tuned to deal with emergencies. However, once you have passed the critical early days following a heart attack and your heart has stabilised, you can use the 'time out' from everyday life to help your body and mind recover from the shock and adjust to the new situation. It is important to take this time.

Aim to offer yourself a stress-free inner world where you free yourself from worries, decisions and difficult emotions. If you sense them coming on, just say, 'I'll look after you when I'm ready. For now I need to rest.' Give yourself permission to do nothing other than allow your heart the maximum care. Say 'no' to too many visitors or noisy radios and televisions.

You may need to follow your natural curiosity about what has happened to you, so when you feel ready to take on new ideas, find out all you can about your heart attack. It may be helpful to ask a friend, partner or family member to write things down for you or be with you when the doctor or consultant is telling you something or explaining a procedure.

While you are in hospital you will have time to rethink your lifestyle. You will probably be given booklets explaining the 'risk factors'. You may have none of them, though this is uncommon. If you do have risk factors, really try hard to use your recovery time positively so that you can start afresh. Resolve to stop smoking, to take more exercise, to lose weight and eat fewer fatty foods, to balance the effort and relaxation periods in your life and to prioritise what is important.

Returning Home

Returning home can be a real treat. And it can be nerve-racking. You might feel anxious about leaving the hospital and your partner might feel the same.

Spend the first period of time just sitting, relaxing, breathing. Then go around your home and check that everything is in its rightful place. Say hello to it all and feel the comfort of the familiarity.

If you live alone, this may be a time when you are convalescing in a nursing home or with friends and relatives. Allow yourself to be looked after as well as taking responsibility for your own medication, rest, exercise programme and diet.

Many hospitals now run a post-heart attack cardiac rehabilitation programme with input from doctors, specialist heart nurses, physiotherapists, occupational therapists and counsellors/psychologists. They are well worth investing the time in joining. Studies have shown that patients who have taken part benefit both physically and psychologically. Alternatively, there may be a community cardiac rehabilitation programme or a support group in your area. Ask the doctor looking after you or phone a national organisation for a group near you (*see Resources, page 251*).

Women, particularly older women, may not be referred for hospital cardiac rehabilitation or not vigorously encouraged to attend. However, real benefits are apparent, especially in older women who often have a considerably lower exercise capacity before the rehabilitation programme, so it is worth asking whether you can take part in one.

Returning to Physical Activity

After heart attacks some people fail to resume their previous level of activity or do not return to work even though they are physically able so to do. This may be because they wrongly believe that there is little hope for them after a heart attack. In fact physical activity will help the heart. After the recovery period from his heart attack of 1977 John began swimming. He built up to a quarter of a mile a day over a period of 18 months and maintained this daily practice. The vessels of his left ventricle were sufficiently strengthened for him not to need surgical intervention for nine years.

Many people wonder how soon they can resume sexual intercourse after a heart attack. If you can walk up two flights of stairs without feeling breathless, it is reasonable to return to sexual activity. It is best to start slowly, initially perhaps taking a more passive role and enjoying the more gentle sensual aspects of love-making. Some partners are nervous about resuming sexual activity for fear of it bringing on another heart attack. There needs to be a shared balance in resuming love-making so that both partners gain the benefits of physical intimacy without compromising the heart. The early months after a heart event are not the time to prove anything, although this may be a strong desire. Sexual activity needs to be built up slowly, in the same way as other physical activities. GTN taken immediately beforehand may help. Sometimes the beta blockers which many people take after a heart attack can cause impotence. If you think this may be happening, talk to your doctor. If you have had a bypass graft it may be best to wait about a month before resuming sexual activity, as the sternum is quite uncomfortable for a while and the extra time will give all the surgery more chance to heal. It is best if you resume sexual activity with your usual partner, as it does appear that the extra *frisson* of a new or extra-relationship partner may put you at more risk.

In scientific terms the level of cardiac exertion for an activity can be expressed as the metabolic turnover of oxygen, or MET. One MET refers to the average energy used per minute while in the resting state, performing activities such as watching television or reading a book. The following table compares the exertion required for sexual activity with that needed for more mundane activities such as housework and walking a mile in 20 minutes.

Activity	MET score/min
Sexual intercourse with long-standing partner	
Normal/lower range	2–3
Vigorous activity/upper range	5–6
Lifting and carrying shopping/heavy objects (9–20 kg)	4–5
Walking a mile in 20 minutes	3–4
Golf	4–5
Gardening	3–5
DIY, wallpapering, etc.	4–5
Light housework, e.g. ironing, polishing	2–4
Heavy housework, e.g. making beds, cleaning windows	3–6
Cycling	4–6

You can fly in an aircraft about two to three weeks after a heart attack. The main problem with flying is not the aircraft but the long corridors associated with airports and the handling of heavy luggage. If you need to fly, arrange with the airline to have a passenger buggy and get someone else to move the baggage.

You can usually drive four weeks after a heart attack. But avoid stressful inner-city traffic.

If you feel worried about resuming physical activity, then it really helps to let the rehabilitation team know this so that specific counselling can be arranged.

Returning to Work

Most people make a full recovery from a heart attack and can return to work. Sometimes angina occurs which needs to have further investigations or water pills are needed because the heart pump is not vigorous enough.

Some people do get seriously depressed after a heart attack and may need treatment but most people recover their equilibrium, although it does take some time. Going back to work may help you recover your self-esteem. Return to work gradually and be vigilant to your emotional needs and levels of stress. (*See* Chapters 3, 16 and 17 for more information on managing stress.)

Remember that you are allowed to stop, breathe and take some space rather than allow yourself to become stressed or upset.

BETTY

Betty was 53 when she had her first heart attack. It came out of the blue, though Betty's family tree shows a pattern of early deaths from heart attack on both her mother's and her father's side. Betty had her first bypass four years after her heart attack and a second five years after that because the grafts had furred up again. Betty's husband had had heart attacks and bypasses and her only son had had a bypass at age 38 and tragically died from a massive coronary ten days after Betty's own repeat bypass. Betty said:

I did go to pieces then. I couldn't stop crying. I was so

> afraid; I wouldn't go out, just sat in a chair and curled up. I was so worried that I was going to have another heart attack, as it hadn't been long since the other operation. My doctor sent me to a wonderful counsellor and she got me through. If I was really down I could phone her and she would talk to me.
>
> This went on for two years. Then I broke my leg and was in plaster and I think the strain of this gave me another heart attack. The doctors decided I needed another bypass. I was worried about this, but I was able to talk to my counsellor about it and she gave me some relaxation and breathing exercises. I did them religiously. Whenever I felt I was tensing up I would go and lie on the bed and do them. I was so tense, it was ages and ages before I could sit without my jaws clamping up. But gradually I found I was able to go out and I didn't curl up in the chair.

Slowly Betty began to learn to live again.

> My opinion is that if the doctors have done so much for you the least you can do is to do as they tell you or as they advise you. Emotions do affect the heart. Expressing your feelings does make the heart hurt, but you've got to talk about them, you mustn't keep them in. Part of the advice I was given was not to hold it back – it's part of the healing.

Betty now keeps herself well through her own programme of self-help as well as medication. She watches her diet, exercises and rather than dwelling on the past keeps herself busy, taking the positive attitude to enjoy life while it lasts.

Angina

Angina is a pain in the chest that usually occurs during exercise or excitement when the heart is called upon to work harder and produce more blood flow. All patients who suffer with angina, whatever its origin, have the burden of pain around their heart and its associated limitation, anxiety and fear. All have to find a way to be with this pain that is, in an overall sense, manageable.

There is an old story about a well-known healer from Europe who went to Africa and met a man who was 150 years old. 'May I ask you a question?' said the healer. 'Of course,' answered the man. 'Tell me, you are 150 years old, do you still feel pain?' The man smiled. 'Of course,' he replied, 'but it does not hurt so much.'

Recognising the Signs

The ideal management for angina is not to allow pain to develop, but to get to know your own body so well that you can sense the triggers for pain and act before they grow into anything major.

There is sometimes a pre-signalling process to angina such as a tickle, itchiness in the chest, harder breathing, general weakness or intuitive flash. The minute this occurs:

♦ Sit down and practise abdominal breathing (*see page 211*) while you focus your mind on a positive image – maybe water, a flower or a green field.

♦ Imagine the vessels around your heart becoming relaxed, wider and full of life-giving blood. Imagine the walls of the blood vessels relaxing, becoming rubbery and flexible, and the blood flowing through – enough 'for boars and birds'!

♦ Stay calm. Panic and fear increase the effort of the heart, raising pulse and blood pressure and stimulating neuro-endochrine arousal. This accentuates and prolongs the pain.

♦ Take glycerine trinitrate (GTN), if necessary, in spray or pill form, just under the tongue.

Self-monitoring

This can also help the management of angina. Writing down when the pain occurs helps you see if there is a pattern to the situations which bring on angina. This can help you to know in advance which situations are likely to be the most demanding upon your energy.

Fatigue will also make you more vulnerable to angina. Use the effort map (*see page 43*) daily in order to ascertain how much energy you have for the tasks you want to do.

Many people live extremely full lives within the limits imposed by angina. They become like experienced mountaineers who, in order to get to the top of the mountain, do not allow themselves to be rushed from behind. Successful mountaineers find a slow, regular pace that matches the available energy to the effort needed to reach the goal, however long it takes. And they get there safely in the end.

Chapter 13

BEFORE AND AFTER CARDIAC SURGERY

My heart aches, and a drowsy numbness
Pains my sense, as though of hemlock I had drunk.

JOHN KEATS, *Ode to a Nightingale*

Being admitted into hospital for any surgical procedure means we have to get used to a strange environment and a constantly changing team of professionals whose jobs we have never heard of before, while often feeling homesick for our familiar 'safe' places! As well as the newness of the sensations and adjusting to hospital routine, noise and smell, we have the experience of things being done to us. If you are able, it is really helpful to have prior information about what to expect, to have done some reading and to have had your questions answered. This chapter will address preparation for and recovery from surgical procedures.

Preparation for Surgery

If you are given a date for surgery and have time for preparation, this is very helpful. If you are an emergency admission, you may only have a few hours to prepare yourself. However much time you have, there are always things you can do.

♦ The first one is – guess! – *breathe*. Practise the breathing techniques recommended throughout this book (*see pages 50 and 211*). They will help you gain the maximum stillness in your body and mind, and allow you to send peace and a smile to the part of your body that is hurting. Partners and family members will also benefit from breathing practice.

♦ The second thing you can do is to focus on *calming your feelings*. First, recognise what they are – probably fear, apprehension, anxiety – and then imagine them to be a storm at sea into which you send a calm and gentle wind.

♦ The third thing you can do is to invite your imagination to work for you. This involves either the visualisation exercises described below or the making of an audiotape based upon the voice of someone you love or someone who has a healing quality and images that are peaceful and restorative for you.

If you have the benefit of time you may also make other preparations. The aim is to get your body into as fit a state as possible for the major adventure it is about to undergo. This is your individual marathon and preparation needs to be no less vigorous.

The shorthand rules are:

♦ Get rested.

♦ Get fit.

♦ Get your mind and emotions in balance.

Get Rested

Make a plan that in the two weeks before the operation you rest or sleep every afternoon and go to bed straight after supper in the evening. Do not take on anything new at work or at home. Tie up loose ends as far as you can or delegate them to other people.

Get Fit

Check out with your doctor how much exercise you can do. Then check with your body how much exercise it feels able to do. Continue with your familiar exercise routine as prescribed by your doctor or cardiac fitness instructor. This may involve floor exercises, weights, walking, swimming or bicycling.

As you rest and exercise, try and focus on the rhythm of *rest and effort* that your body needs. Some days your body may not want to do much; other days it will wish to be stretched. *Use your body as your guide – always ask it first.*

Get Your Mind and Emotions in Balance

Spend this time with people you love and in exchanges that are good for the heart in the emotional and spiritual sense. Make your meditation or mindfulness practice a bit longer each day. Say special prayers that are important for you; make special pilgrimages to those holy places that mean something to your spiritual heart. Try and focus on asking open-heartedly for the strength to be present with whatever is to pass.

Self-hypnosis and Visualisation

In his book *Healing from the Heart,* leading cardiovascular surgeon Mehmet Oz writes about the research trials at New York's Colombia Presbyterian Medical Center which asked the question: 'Can self-hypnosis and visualisation therapy help patients get through surgery?'

The trials involved two groups of heart disease patients – those who used self-hypnosis and visualisation tapes during surgery and those who did not. They found that patients taught self-hypnosis had lower scores for fatigue. Interestingly, the worst outcomes came in the group that was taught self-hypnosis but did not follow the instructions.

It is interesting to speculate here that being active in all your involvements with your health is the key. Those of us who want a 'magic bullet' to take away our suffering and who project that magic bullet on to others in terms of what they expect become passive, less responsible and therefore more prone to disappointment.

In another study, the Greenleaf Fisher study at the Albert Einstein College of Medicine in New York in the 1990s, patients formed three groups: one with no self-hypnosis training; one with training and the suggestion that they relaxed and imagined themselves as floppy rag dolls or bean bags to allow muscle relaxation; and one with training and the instruction to focus upon six specific areas, including keeping blood pressure comfortable, letting defence systems stay alert before, during and after surgery, cooperating with treatment by flowing along with procedures, and looking forward to a quick return to normal bodily functions and a lifestyle free of pain and fear. The self-hypnosis training was given one or two days before surgery. After surgery, the investigators monitored the patients' blood pressure, wound drainage and length of time on the respirator. The patients in the two self-hypnosis groups recovered faster in the first 48 hours after surgery than the other patients.

● PRE-SURGICAL VISUALISATION

This is an exercise we designed for patients.

● Sit comfortably with your back supported and your eyes closed.

● Concentrate upon your breathing ... regular, slow in-breaths and out-breaths ... for a few minutes.

● Allow your thoughts to wander in and out... Don't let a thought get a hold on your energy. If a thought comes, just recognise it and let it go.

● Breathe in and become aware of your heart.

● Breathe out and smile to your heart.

- Breathe in and become aware of your heart.

- Breathe out and imagine your heart being held and supported by kind hands.

- Stay with this image as you allow your breathing to become automatically slow ... and regular.

- As your heart is being held and supported in kind hands, imagine that your whole body is held safely in a beautiful place. It may be a place that you know and love or a place that is offered to you now in your imagination. Feel the soft fabric beneath you, covering and protecting you; smell the pure fragrances ... pine, lavender, rose, sandalwood; hear the sounds dearest to you ... music, birdsong, the soft breeze ...

- Imagine a source of great light, the light of many concentrated points of healing, that is beaming in to this sacred space.

- Spend some time allowing the sounds, smells and atmosphere of this place to hold and support you, and the light to bathe you in its balm.

- Now imagine the kind hands beginning to mend the suffering in your arteries and heart in this protected and beautiful space. Offer them your concentrated effort, your energy, your good-will. Imagine the blood beginning to flow through the restored vessels, the pressure in the vessel walls beginning to relax, to allow the flow of life-giving blood to be smooth and clear, and to spread itself around your entire body. Imagine receiving oxygen through the lungs into the blood now being pumped around the heart, and that oxygen serving all the organs of your body.

- Imagine now that your heart is mended, restored, given new promise of life. Imagine it happily folded into the heartcloth inside the nest of the chest wall protected by the ribcage, beating strongly and firmly with the heartbeat of your life.

- Allow your breathing to relax now with the sense of your own heartbeat nearby and know that all is well.

Hospital Admission

Admission into hospital for surgery has its own unique procedures involving lots of paperwork, the taking of blood and urine samples, checking past medical and surgical details and the taking of the names and addresses of your nearest and dearest. These processes are routine and offer a way of getting you orientated in the hospital environment. If you have never been in hospital before it can be strange and unnerving. But you will be asked the same questions over and over again and even though this can be irritating, it is a way of getting in there!

You may be able to have some of your own things with you, such as photographs or special texts. These can be a vital link to what is closest to you when visitors have gone and you are on your own.

Knowledge is Power

Knowing what procedures are going to take place and what will happen to you as a patient gives you some clarity and power within what can be a helpless situation. As a patient you are allowed to know and to ask questions so that you have this clarity. It helps to have someone with you who can also hear what medical staff are saying.

It is also immensely helpful to have a notebook in which you have written details of past medical or surgical events and the medications you are currently taking. This is also a good place to write down anything you want to know more about. So often when we are asked whether there is anything we want to know we go blank. If you have a notebook with you, you will not be lost for words. Your notebook is a good friend.

Some people also use their notebooks as a kind of diary to record events and feelings. I often use mine to record thoughts, sayings or ideas that come into my head, especially in new and strange environments. You might also use your notebook to write down your dreams. These can offer us remarkable insights.

Relationships with Medical and Surgical Staff

Being able to establish a rapport with the medical team that is going to look after you is helpful and reassuring. It is important to try and secure a good feeling and trust.

John Wallwork, a cardiothoracic surgeon and head of the transplant team at Papworth Hospital, says: 'It is essential to see the person beforehand and I spend all day relating patients' disease to their lives and what they do .... Doctors used to talk *to* patients whereas now they talk *with* patients. If I were going to have a heart operation, the most useful thing would be for someone to treat me like an intelligent person who didn't know the answers. I would not want to be patronised.'

Complications

Part of preparation is also to speak to someone close to you of what you wish for in the unlikely event of complications. While it is unlikely that anything will go wrong because heart surgery is well established and the risks are low, nevertheless unexpected events do occur that are beyond anyone's control. It is important that your wishes are known, both for you and, particularly, for those family members who may have to make decisions on your behalf when you are unconscious. This is particularly true for young people whose parents will take some responsibility, but it is a relief for all concerned to have an idea of the patient's wishes if the time were to come when those wishes needed to be honoured. (*See also page 196.*)

After Surgery

After major surgery it is natural to feel shocked and even depressed, especially after surgery involving the heart, which is the most potent of organs. Many patients feel tearful – some from an overwhelming sense of relief that the operation is over and that they are alive. Some people feel grateful and their heart is full. Others feel angry and resentful for having to have a heart operation, especially if they have none of the assumed risk factors and 'Why me?' is their uppermost thought. Some feel gloomy about recovery and returning to the life they had before. All these feelings and thoughts may be rushing through your mind in the early days following heart surgery.

In the days immediately after an operation some people suffer from psychological disturbances such as mood swings – feeling 'high' or manic one minute and extremely down the next. Some people suffer from nightmares and anxiety. These responses are thought to be connected to being on the heart-lung bypass machine (probably due to microemboli created by the heart-lung machine going to the brain). In most patients these disturbances pass after ten days. Even symptoms that seem to hang about, such as moodiness, difficulty in concentrating and depressed thinking, have usually gone after three months.

On returning home, some people feel anxious or depressed, or feel that they are not making as much progress as they should. These feelings are frequent after any major surgery once your normal impatience begins to assert itself. Although from day to day your progress may seem slow, it will improve over time. Learning to develop patience with yourself and your efforts is all part of respecting your body and what it has been through. Patience is of huge importance for the development of stamina and the future care of the heart.

Coronary Artery Bypass Grafting

What happens in coronary artery bypass grafting is that a bypass graft is created to take blood from the aorta to the coronary artery past where the narrowing or blockage is found. This may be a vein from the leg, or sometimes an artery from the arm, which can be used without interfering with the health of the arm. Increasingly, surgeons are using an artery that runs inside the chest wall. This is called the internal mammary artery and using it appears to be better than using leg veins in some patients. The internal mammary artery graft appears to last longer than a vein graft, probably because it was originally designed to take arterial pressure. As a result most people will have an internal mammary graft and one or two vein grafts. The surgeon needs to operate on the heart when it is not working so a heart-lung machine takes over the role of circulating blood round the body for the time that the surgeon is performing the operation. (There is now an operation that is done on the beating heart – called 'minimally invasive' surgery – but it is only suitable for narrowings of a particular artery, the left anterior descending, and then only when there is disease just in this artery.)

Coronary artery bypass grafting is tremendously successful and the risk of dying from it is less than 2 per cent. Certain conditions increase the risk, such as poor pump (ventricular) function and disease of the main left coronary artery (left main stem stenosis). Diabetes also makes the operation more difficult as arteries are often smaller.

The operation does not cure the condition or the underlying problems, but is an elegant way of relieving the main symptom of chest pain. About 80 per cent of people experience complete relief from pain after the operation and this may last for a long time. About 5 per cent of patients get pain back each year as the underlying disease progresses.

The hospital stay is usually about six to nine days; patients are often in the critical or intensive care unit for 24 hours, or longer if there are complications. Convalescence should continue for the first week or two and then activity can gradually be increased. Full recovery should occur within about two to three months, although older patients may take longer to recover.

The breastbone or sternum is divided for the operation and this takes some weeks to heal. Coughing with a pillow clutched to the chest may help initially. Sometimes there are pins and needles or numbness from the site where the leg vein has been; this should not cause concern. There may also be some swelling of the leg on that side, but elastic support stockings and keeping the leg elevated for a few weeks after the operation should deal with this. (Minimally invasive surgery does not require the sternum to be cut.)

Recovery from Coronary Artery Bypass Grafting

♦ You can usually drive six weeks after a bypass operation.

♦ You should probably wait four weeks after a bypass operation before resuming sexual intercourse.

♦ Continue taking aspirin long term.

♦ Think about returning to work two to three months after the operation.

As mentioned above, short-term psychological problems are common after surgery and usually pass. Although some people claim poor concentration and memory loss after a bypass graft, studies have in fact shown that these patients actually need counselling for emotional problems and that their difficulties are emotional at base.

Psychological counselling or therapy can offer a vital space for the naming and understanding of any emotional difficulties experienced. These problems may well be rooted in the past and have surfaced more profoundly after surgery. A good therapist will be able to make an assessment of those difficulties that stem from earlier attitudes and offer help with those that arise from the operation itself. In all cases, finding a way to live confidently with the fact of heart surgery, its implications for the future, its limitations for the present and all its many individual meanings, is an important part of recovery.

Some people may have intermittent impotence problems following bypass, and defects in the visual field may occur in some individuals, resulting from the bypass procedure.

Valve Replacement Surgery

We saw earlier that open heart surgery has revolutionised the treatment of faulty valves and that there are two types of replacement valve: the tissue type, which lasts 15 to 20 years, and the metal type, which lasts indefinitely (*see page 119*). Metal valve replacement involves the taking of Warfarin because of clotting potential around the valve.

The surgical procedures for a replacement valve operation are the same as for the bypass operation except that the operation does not take as long. The chest has to be opened via the sternum and the recovery follows along similar lines to the bypass operation (*see above*).

Heart Transplant

Once, patients whose hearts were so diseased or damaged they could not be repaired could only be offered pain relief and oxygen. Then, in 1967, the very first heart transplant was performed in South Africa by Christiaan Barnard. Today in Britain about 300 transplant operations are carried out annually at eight centres around the country. The reason for heart transplants is end stage coronary artery disease, which may be associated with severe heart failure, cardiomyopathy or congenital heart disease.

While waiting for a donor heart, there are many devices and procedures that may support the damaged heart system. People in the UK who go on to a transplant list to await a donor heart usually have a 50/50 risk of dying within a year from very severe heart failure. The average waiting time once on the list is six months. The physical implications of subjecting an already ill person to complex surgery are great and patients are given thorough screening before going on to the transplant list.

The support offered by the heart transplant team is tremendous. They are there from the time the patient goes on to the list right through the surgery and the post-operative period to the rehabilitation phase. It can be a tense time waiting for a donor heart, especially with the added awareness that another person has to die in order to give you the opportunity of a new life. All the transplant patients I have met personally, or read about, wished to offer their gratitude to the individual donor and to the families who had given permission for another life to go on at their time of greatest loss. Physicians, surgeons, physiotherapists, nurse therapists and counsellors will all be ready to help you and your family with the many practical as well as physical and psychological needs.

After surgery there is often a period of balancing medication and waiting to ensure that the new heart becomes familiar with its new body and is not rejected. There are stories about the cell memory of the donor's heart transmitting data from its former owner to the new owner. New research studies (Paul Pearsall and Candace Pert in the United States) have suggested that there is much more to memory than we have previously known. These studies contain data which is challenging for the morality and philosophy of transplantation, and fascinating for cell biologists and psychologists, and it is clear that we need much more data in order to understand the phenomenon more clearly. Most importantly, professionals looking after terminally ill heart patients who have been given a donor heart need to be able to offer as much psychological and emotional care as possible.

Artificial Hearts

There are several devices that help a patient waiting for a transplant who is too ill to be at home because their heart needs constant support. These devices are more commonly used in the USA than in the UK. One is the LVAD (the Left Ventricular Assist Device), a mechanical pump the size of a CD player. It is fascinating to record that this mechanical device inspired cardiothoracic surgeon Mehmet Oz in New York to pioneer complementary approaches such as homoeopathy and massage therapy, and also to understand the growth of stem cells.

Another artificial heart is the Jarvik 2000 pump, a tiny battery-operated turbine that can be implanted into the left ventricle of the heart to propel oxygenated blood around the body. The first person to have this device permanently implanted was a British hospital psychotherapist, Peter Houghton, at the John Radcliffe Hospital in Oxford. He had been given just a few weeks to live and had resigned himself to this fate. However, by the chance intervention of a friend, he was offered the opportunity to make medical history by having the mini-heart implanted. After initial problems with infection and pain, he is now able to walk again and is coming to terms with having extra time he had not prepared for.

The use of the artificial heart is not yet operational in cardiothoracic units in Britain, but more trials are under way.

BRIAN AND ANNA

I meet Anna soon after John was admitted to Papworth Hospital critical care unit. Her husband Brian had had a successful heart and lung transplant operation the day before and now Anna had the job of telephoning all their relatives to let them know the news. Later Brian wrote:

> I didn't know I had a problem with my heart until I had an assessment for a lung transplant and was told they would have to do a heart and lung transplant as my heart was damaged and would not stand a major operation. I had suffered from bronchiectasis for several years, which means that my heart had to work harder to get air to my lungs. I was on oxygen for up to 24 hours a day before the operation. I spent most of my day sitting in the chair and my wife had to put my socks on for me.
>
> Feeling part of a social group and being able to express feeling affect the heart. My family and friends have been and still are a tower of strength for me and the medical staff at my local hospital and Papworth Hospital

are magnificent. Feelings such as joy, love and happiness all help me to feel at ease and I breathe nice and easy. Feelings such as loneliness and sadness make my breathing laboured; worrying and frustration make my heart beat faster, while hurt makes my heart feel heavy and labouring.

Brian has made a fantastic recovery since his transplant. He walks over a mile each day, does regular breathing exercises and takes the regular compulsory medication. He and Anna have been on three holidays abroad – making up for lost time! There have been adjustments emotionally as well as physically. They have both had their 'low' times after the operation, and Anna has had to adjust to her role as helper.

Brian says that the most surprising thing about his experience was the speed with which he recovered his health:

I feel as if I have been reborn, only 10 years younger. What I would say to other people is to *never* give up hope, and if you are lucky enough to be offered the chance of a transplant, don't be afraid to take it.

Chapter 14

COPING WITH INTENSIVE CARE

History is filled with examples that demonstrate how human contact acts as one of nature's most powerful antidotes to stress.

DR JAMES LYNCH, *The Broken Heart*

O PEN HEART SURGERY is always followed by at least 24 hours in intensive care. Patients who have had a heart transplant or heart and lung transplant tend to be nursed intensively for longer, as their bodies are carefully monitored for signs of rejecting the new tissues. Heart patients spending time in intensive care may also include those suffering from acute cardiomyopathy after a virus; those who are waiting for a donor heart and those who have suffered complications to their surgery, such as pneumonia or stroke.

Patterns of recovery are individual and depend upon prior conditions such as diabetes, lung capacity and responses to the shock and invasion of surgery. However well prepared, however skilled a surgical team, there is always the chance of an unexpected event.

Some patients need longer than others to recover after surgery and to be ready to be discharged to the ward. Although intensive care staff are keen to discharge patients from intensive care as soon as possible, because of the risk of infection, disorientation and institutionalisation, patients need to be able to take the next step into more independent recovery without the support of ventilation and intensity of monitoring.

Some patients become 'long-stay patients' who do not make it through the first available 'window' of opportunity, such as coming off ventilation, maintaining an upward pattern of getting well, but suffer complications such as infection, stroke or breathing difficulties.

However, patients can survive three or four months of intensive care and live to walk out weakened but able to get well eventually. Success rate for first bypass surgery is 98 per cent, with the risk of complication increasing in second bypass surgery to 4 per cent. Risk in valve replacement surgery is 1 per cent, rising to 4 per cent for valve replacement plus coronary artery bypass grafting.

It is sobering to reflect that while seeing one's loved one in intensive care is painful, if they were not in that place at that time, they would be dead. To witness a relative in intensive care, to see them beginning to recover and enter life again, and then to see them walking in the garden at home or even playing sport is a moving and fantastic miracle. And it is this latter image that is the predominant outcome.

The Experience of Intensive Care

Many hospitals now offer patients and their partners a glimpse of the inside of an intensive care unit before planned surgery, as a way of preparation. Patients are at liberty to request this opportunity. It is useful in terms of knowing visually what to expect from a room and of gaining some idea of protocol. Nothing can really prepare a patient for the actual experience, both physical and emotional, of waking up on ventilation surrounded by bleeping equipment. Equally, nothing can prepare relatives for seeing their loved one lying unconscious surrounded by the tubes, drains and drips, with medical and surgical technology beeping away, knowing that their life is largely dependent upon those brilliant inventions. But if you have seen the intensive care unit beforehand, you will be more prepared.

Intensive care units are extraordinary places. They contain the extremes – pure clinical excellence and pure human love. The specialist machines monitor every bodily function. Portable X-ray machines and blood testing laboratories are nearby. They are staffed by highly qualified, dedicated professionals – nurses, doctors, anaesthetists, surgeons, physiotherapists, X-ray technicians – who support every aspect of the life in their hands. This team is managed by a consultant intensivist whose speciality is intensive care medicine. It really is intense, hence the name, and it is a very different experience from the ward.

Most hospitals provide their intensive care patients with one nurse per patient for the entirety of their shift. Many nurses have told me that they like this long period because it helps them to get to know their patient and to bond with them. This is particularly needed because the patient is usually unconscious or severely ill. Every bodily function is monitored – fluid intake by drip feed, fluid output by catheter for urine into a bag attached to the rail underneath the bed and by drains and bags for scar tissue fluids. Heart rate, blood pressure and oxygen input data are available on a television screen which also prints out the ECG; blood gases are taken every 15 minutes in the early post-operative stages to check for oxygen levels. Patients are 'intubated' and put on ventilation – a plastic tube is inserted into the lungs via the mouth and breathing is done by mechanical pump. The machine gradually reduces the number of 'breaths' so that the patient slowly gets used to taking their own breaths until they are ready to be free of the breathing tube completely and can breathe on their own.

This post-operative period is a crucial time and medical staff will be carefully monitoring the body's immediate response to the trauma of surgery. The first major event occurs when the patient is invited to cough and expel the ventilator tube and breathe unaided. When this is successful it is a relief to the patient, who no longer has the discomfort of the tube going into their airway. Patients who are slower to return to consciousness will take longer to expel the tube, but it usually comes out as soon as possible to minimise the risk of infection. When natural breathing is established, fluid input and output is regulated, blood gases are satisfactory and consciousness returned, the patient is taken to the ward.

Intensive care is usually very warm and heart surgery patients lie naked except for one sheet so that their chests are available. Women, who are in the minority, are covered to protect their modesty. In a hospital where cardiac surgery is performed, it is a common morning sight to see a growing row of middle-aged men with vivid chest scars lying prone and on ventilation, having undergone their bypass operations. The next day they have gone to the ward and the next row of patients is getting ready to file in.

Post-operative Responses and Complications

Emergencies can happen suddenly in intensive care – cardiac or pulmonary arrest, stroke, bleeding, loss of consciousness and death. The staff are all highly trained to deal with both the repetitive intimacy of intensive care, for which a great deal of patience and attention to minute detail are required, and with the emergencies that can and do occur.

Post-operatively, complications occur when natural breathing is not able to be restored due to poor coronary output or chest infection, or when neurological events have compromised breathing and recovery function. These may include stroke – caused when a blood clot forms in the brain or when the brain receives insufficient oxygen during surgery due to a drop in blood pressure or complications of surgery necessitating longer time on the heart bypass machine.

Patients may also need kidney dialysis if their urine output is continually poor, indicating that the kidneys' function has been compromised.

Tracheostomy

If a patient is still too weak to breathe unaided and it is considered that they have been on ventilation long enough, a tracheostomy is performed. The procedure takes place under anaesthetic. A small tube is inserted into the throat leading down the windpipe into the lungs. It has a rim around it so that ventilation equipment may be attached and protection may be added during eating so that food does not get into the windpipe. This means that patients may be attached to a ventilator and also learn to breathe on their own. Their mouth is freed, so they find it easier to swallow and eat and can kiss their family and friends! A tracheostomy tube can be a good friend and some people have them for a very long time while they are healing.

Resuscitation

Sometimes a patient moves swiftly into a critical or emergency situation where medical staff have to ask immediately about resuscitation. If your loved one has been admitted into intensive care it is useful to spend some time writing down the kinds of question that might come up.

It is important to check your hospital's policy on resuscitation – whether a patient will receive this automatically or whether there might be a policy of DNR, 'Do Not Resuscitate'. Every hospital is different. (It is also important to realise that a DNR decision, especially on a general ward, is not about withdrawing care or treatments such as antibiotics but a decision about whether the heart or brain will survive the resuscitation.)

Decisions about resuscitation must involve the next of kin and be based upon medical facts and concerns, quality of life and suffering, and the wishes of the patient, which may or may not be known. The consultant intensivist is in charge of these decisions.

I (Elizabeth) was encouraged by my own experience of intensive care at Papworth Hospital, whose policy was to treat the whole patient. The intensive care speciality was to support what each patient could do in response to their individual treatment, thus meeting the patient's needs. For example, oxygen can be reduced to see how much oxygen a patient can create by themselves. It is equally so with drugs such as dopamine that support the heart's function. Each day the team assesses how the patient is responding to treatment.

When the unit is having to give more and more oxygen, drugs and treatments, thus literally 'keeping the body going by machine', the consultant will speak to the next of kin. Decisions about further treatment can emerge healthily and helpfully from these shared discussions. They are painful and difficult discussions and require everyone involved to stretch their thinking to the utmost. Keeping a notebook of past treatment, the issues raised by this and questions to ask, as well as having the fruits of discussions with wise friends and elders, friends or priests can help during these times. Everyone will be individual in their response to intensive care treatment, whether they demand the team to do everything possible to keep their loved one alive or whether a decision has to be made that all that can be done has been done and the person should be allowed to die with dignity, free of pain.

Post-intensive Care Difficulties

Most short-stay patients in intensive care do not remember much about the experience. The most common complaints are about the noise, the heat and the lack of a sense of time passing. Many units have responded to these complaints as best they can by having windows so that patients may have a sense of day and night, of sky, even trees and birds, and by turning down the overhead lights at night.

For longer-stay patients in intensive care, the most

common physical problems are severe weakness, stiffness of joints and fatigue. Two per cent of muscle mass is lost per day and over a long time patients may lose half their muscle mass, requiring a long period of rebuilding through physiotherapy. When muscle mass is reduced, it affects the cough muscles, so that the power of cough is reduced, with less control over swallowing and taking in food satisfactorily.

Memory and concentration may be poor after intensive care, which can be frustrating and lead to feelings of depression and irritability. The need for morale boosting is paramount. Small, manageable tasks should be arranged according to the energy available.

Longer periods in intensive care may also induce a temporary dependence or institutionalisation and patients may feel fearful of leaving their protected environment. Their families, too, may feel nervous about their being in the less intensely staffed ward and fearful of having to take responsibility for them later on at home. The surgical ward nursing staff should be able to help here and many patients go home with a telephone number they can ring to talk to a staff nurse if problems should occur.

Some patients report startling dreams and nightmares while in intensive care, largely induced by medication and lack of continuous sleep, and there are even incidences of post-traumatic stress disorder in those who have had a prolonged and frightening experience of being in intensive care. These cases are the rare minority for heart patients. Largely, their time in intensive care will quickly pass into memory and they will be able to get on with their lives.

Support for Relatives

It is easy for relatives to feel alarmed to see their loved one lying helpless, shocked, drugged and on a life-support machine. Relatives need all the support they can get for their vigil with their loved one during this time. This means physical support in terms of somewhere to stay, in the hospital or nearby, regular small meals and lots of hot drinks, the helping hands of friends, relatives to sit with, the psychological support of staff and doctors who can give information to clear fears and fantasies, and something to do that will help hold concentration and maintain stamina.

While intensive care units are busy places with focused care and lots of machinery and technical skill, I have found them to be extremely caring. Nurses are the key. As already mentioned, a patient will often have a special nurse for the day, with whom you can talk and discuss progress. This is very helpful, as you can begin to get a real feel for what is going on from one person rather than hearing lots of different approaches from different staff.

Every hospital will have its own policy on visitors, but as a rule relatives can visit an intensive care patient any time they wish. Entry into the unit is always by way of a bell, to allow staff to protect other patients while giving treatments and to manage their work alongside the needs of relatives. Sitting or standing by your relative, holding their hand and speaking to them helps you to feel you are offering something to a situation where you can easily feel helpless. Research shows that it also affects the patient, whether conscious or unconscious.

There are also times in between when you are unable to go into the intensive care unit or you actually need a break from it yourself. Many relatives spend long hours waiting outside intensive care units while treatment of many different kinds is carried out or while waiting to speak to doctors. There are relatives' rooms, which have often been decorated or furnished with gifts from other grateful relatives who have had to find solace and patience in the midst of pain and distress. Sometimes there is a television there, a pile of magazines, books and even games. I often wondered, during my five-week vigil in intensive care, whether anyone actually was able to focus on anything other than the immediate problem. But relatives need a place to be together to discuss the progress of their loved one. They need a place to sit and think, to weep, to drink endless cups of tea, to pray or meditate, or to gaze out of a window at the trees and sky and wonder at the meaning of life and death.

JOHN MCCORMICK

During the first week of John's time in intensive care our shared six children were with me in one of the small visitors' rooms at Papworth Hospital. Four of the adult children had flown from California, Washington State and Massachusetts, together with a daughter-in-law and new five-month-old granddaughter. Two had travelled from Cornwall and Wales, one pregnant with a new grandson. From time to time other close family members and friends came to join us, cramped into the tiny room.

In the room we placed the flowers sent by friends, John's favourite yellow roses and some photographs of him, and every day we lit a candle. One of us would make a drawing of the 'hope' for the day – oxygen input, fluid output, coming off the balloon pump, being ready to come off ventilation. We sat together.

One by one, occasionally in pairs, we also sat with John, each of us communicating with him in our own personal way. We talked, we cried, we held the baby, we prayed, meditated, we shared stories about the beloved man who was fighting for his life. We imagined him having a near-death experience and returning as a guru in a purple kaftan; we laughed. We found food to eat and bottled drinks to make a change from the inevitable drinks machines. We went out for walks in twos and threes. We joked with black humour; we struggled to understand all the new terminology and the choices the doctors were having to make as they monitored John's every tiny movement. Those vital moments were the last ones we were able to have with him.

The waiting areas are where you also meet the relatives of other patients and share stories. This can be helpful and encouraging. It can be very moving and useful to imagine that at these moments, throughout the world, there are millions of other people in similar situations, bearing witness to the sick and dying. Bearing witness is done for the one and for the many. On a personal and intimate level you also meet other people who are going through their own struggle and drama. It was in the critical care unit that I met Anna, and later Brian, with whom I spent valuable and supportive time.

Meeting other relatives can also be disconcerting. I remember early on after John's surgery hearing that another woman's husband had been there for three weeks and thinking, 'Oh no,' and feeling very fearful. Then, at a later stage, I was asked by another relative whose partner had just undergone surgery and was having problems how long my husband had been there. When I said, 'Two weeks,' she looked horrified.

Advice for Relatives

♦ Try and be truly present. Think only of one hour, one day, at a time. If you find yourself slipping into past or future thinking ('If only...', 'What if...?'), just gently bring your thoughts back to the present.

♦ Think of your loved one as moving only one step at a time.

♦ Keep focusing on the person they are, on what you imagine they would like to hear, how they would like to be touched.

♦ Keep a small notebook and write things down – questions, medical and surgical facts, details of treatment.

♦ Find people you trust to talk to.

♦ Keep eating, drinking, exercising and getting fresh air.

♦ Take short walks outside as often as you can.

♦ Find easy reading.

♦ Find ways to relax, to meditate or pray – not on outcome, but on having the strength to accept whatever happens.

♦ Be kind to yourself.

Support for the Patient

Intensive care units pull us from our everyday world where we don't think very deeply about the meaning of life into intensely sharp areas about life and death – what it is to be human and what we can offer another human being in suffering.

I believe that everything we offer another person has value, whether they are conscious or unconscious. I believe there is a soulful intelligence in each of us that is aware of presence and intent. Speak to the patient, read poetry, news, bring in a Walkman and play their favourite music, stories or talking books. Hold their hand, rub their feet and legs, ask to be allowed to perform some of the nursing duties so that they might be comforted by your touch, your smell, optimism and your positive intent.

JOHN MCCORMICK

John spent three weeks continuously in intensive care after getting pneumonia on the tenth day after his bypass operation and suffering a respiratory arrest from which he was resuscitated. Most of the time he was unconscious or seemingly lost in consciousness. He did not speak, as he was at first on a ventilator, then had a tracheostomy. As I have written above, during this time our collective six children sat with him at different times and told him of their love, as did many other relatives and friends. The constant presence of people who loved John helped to keep the human face of the man whom the nurses had only known as a critically ill patient. This created a bond which supported us all.

Patients who have come through these experiences have spoken of their subliminal experience of receiving an atmosphere of love and positive regard that seemed like a warm blanket of care and support during the harshness of intense treatment. It is the human aspect that often helps people through to wherever they need to go. Never underestimate the connections you can make at any time in any place and under any circumstances.

Chapter 15

COPING WITH DEATH

Give sorrow words, the grief that does not speak
whispers o'er the fraught heart, and bids it break.
WILLIAM SHAKESPEARE, *Macbeth*

IT IS IMPOSSIBLE to write about the heart and not to include death, both for heart patients and for their families to ponder upon. Death from heart disease is common and ultimately death is something we all have to embrace and come to terms with. It is much better to face it than live in fear of it. Once accepted it really is less frightening.

Near-death Experience

Many patients have 'near-death experiences' (NDEs), when they lose consciousness as their heart stops beating and regain consciousness with a profound sense of having been to another place. Many patients do not speak of these experiences for fear of being thought mad; some try to speak to hospital doctors about them and are met with hostility. But near-death studies have been conducted which have concluded that the process of death has a universal pattern:

- A sense of peace and well-being.

- Separation from the body and the world.

- Entering darkness.

- Seeing a light.

- Entering the light.

In Buddhist tradition, the process of entering death is extremely important in order to establish a proper rebirth. Buddhists speak of the need for those closest to the dying person to continue to honour them as they have been in this life, offering gratitude and thanks for all the gifts they brought and wishing them well as they enter the 'bardo', the unknown land that is thought to be where souls live between earthly lives.

One of the most useful aspects of the recording of near-death experiences and the long-held tradition of Buddhist practice is the shift in attitude to death from fearful and negative to hopeful and positive. People who have had near-death experiences do seem to lose their fear of the passage to death and, perhaps because of this, are able to embrace life more freely, with less anxiety and limitation upon their energy. Many people cite their brush with death as their moment of spiritual awakening, an awakening that led to huge changes in their attitude and everyday lives.

Fear of Death

Some people with heart disease fear the potential closeness of death. Others are relieved by the idea that their passage to the next world will be a quick one. Of course, none of us knows the nature of our own death. Death itself is in charge and will come calling when it is time. Much of our fear of death is our fear of not being in control and being in pain. Hospitals and hospice care now offer a great deal of help in the relief of pain in terminal illness, so allowing a person to die more peacefully.

If you feel that not enough medication or help for pain is being given, this needs to be discussed with your doctor.

Death itself is beyond our control. What we can do is be as prepared for death as we can be – both the death of our loved ones and ourselves. Many people find this impossible. Others are helped by their religious or spiritual beliefs about the nature of death and life hereafter.

It takes time to become accustomed to the fact that everyone and everything dies eventually. But rather than avoid the fact of death, which can add to the fear and anxiety surrounding it, it is better to get used to death as being part of life. It may be useful to talk to someone about the different traditions surrounding death and dying. Many of the religious and spiritual traditions are able to offer philosophical support.

It is true that however much we love someone, we cannot keep them alive. And none of us knows how we will feel when a loved one dies and is no longer a warm presence in our every day, however much warning we have about the possibility of their death. But the love we feel is never lost.

If you find yourself becoming fixated upon death in a negative, morbid way it may be connected to a negative experience of death in the past. If these memories have led to you becoming depressed, it would be useful to consult a psychological counsellor.

All heart patients and their families must face the fact of death at any time. Trying not to worry is difficult, and loved ones must learn to manage their own anxiety and not pass it on to those around, especially the patient, who will have fears of their own. I (Elizabeth) found it very hard not to be anxious. If the phone rang at an odd time, my first thought would be: 'Is it John?' This is normal and I had to find ways of living with the anxiety by recognising it as such, often giving myself more time for everyday tasks if I was particularly anxious and being wary of developing the habit of hypervigilance that would then compromise my own health. There were times when I did not have the energy for work and had to ask for my own patients' and colleagues' understanding with this.

It helps to know that if you are supporting all the appropriate changes in lifestyle and attitude that will help improve your loved one's condition and that should they have a heart attack while you are there, you will know what to do (*see page 244*), you have learned all you can. But you cannot prevent a heart attack happening and should it occur anywhere else there is nothing you can do. Learning to live with this knowledge, and the feeling of helplessness this can create, means taking care of your own anxiety and not passing it on. Then the times you have together are as free as possible, and this is the best help. All of us can only do our best, recognise this and forgive ourselves for what we are unable to do.

None of us knows what happens after death and none of us knows, until we experience it, what it will be like to be without someone who is very dear to us. But once we have accepted that death will actually happen and we have a desire for 'good death', either for ourselves or for our loved ones, we are actually freed from the anxiety to control anything and freed to live fully, every moment. We have the opportunity then to experience life as a gift.

Facing Death

People facing their own death need to be able to talk about it if they wish and not talk about it if they do not wish. Making the opportunity is important. It is also important to create the space where fears, hopes and any unfinished business may be aired, as well as share questions about the passage from one life to another.

Having been witness to my own husband John's passage through to death I am convinced that although the body does indeed reach the end of its sustainable life, the spirit does go on. In what form is a mystery, but the energy present at the moment of death and from experience afterwards is palpable – and has even been photographed – and this is enough to convince me that there is something else.

Being present at the moment of death is a privilege. But even if you are not able to be present physically, by having decided to open your heart to the process of death you have chosen to be present. Being with someone you love in heart and spirit is what is truly most important. We may not be able to be present with their actual body, but on the energetic levels that go beyond the limitations of physical awareness, if we can be truly with the other person's spirit as they leave this world, that experience will be shared.

PART FIVE

Keeping Your Heart Healthy

Chapter 16

BREATHING, EXERCISE AND DIET

When we touch beneath the busyness of thought, we discover a sweet healing silence, an inherent peacefulness in each of us, a goodness of heart, strength, and wholeness that is our birthright.

JACK KORNFIELD, *A Path with Heart*

THE HEART IS such a marvellous piece of equipment. It is the strongest muscle in the body and also the most sensitive. This sensitivity means that the heart is highly responsive to our efforts on its behalf.

In respect and support of our heart, it is our task to be truly mindful of all that we ask it to do for us. We assist the heart's physical function by releasing all the energy we can for it to do its own healing work. We have seen in earlier chapters that the 'hardening down' of emotions such as fear and anger and the reverberations of anxiety and long-term depression affect the physical heart. The best medicine we can offer the heart is to learn to be present with everything that happens to us at any time and to breathe consciously into the experience.

Breathing

There are two different practices involving breathing that we suggest for daily use.

1. Abdominal breathing

This is breathing from the belly, which will help you to use the entire chest cavity. This will mean that all the cells and muscles in your body – including your heart – will benefit from the nourishing flow of oxygen. Abdominal breathing also helps you to feel a greater spaciousness inside, instead of the cramped feeling that so often accompanies heart difficulties. Its value as a support is that it can be practised anywhere at any time.

The practice helps you to avoid building up stress or getting into the habit of hyperventilation. You may find it helpful to learn this kind of breathing from a teacher – a yoga, relaxation or Alexander Technique practitioner (*see page 236*) or a singer.

- Sit with your back straight, or lie down flat with just a slim pillow to support your head.

- Place one hand on your upper abdomen (in the region of your solar plexus).

- Practise pushing these muscles in and out so that you can feel them working. (It might take time to get used to this if you have not been aware of your diaphragm.)

- Relax your shoulders and put your other hand on your upper chest. As you breathe normally, notice which hand moves the most.

The In-breath
The in-breath draws in the oxygen that keeps us alive.

On the in-breath, practise pushing the abdomen out, so that the diaphragm descends to expand the base of your lungs. It might feel strange at first, but keep persevering. If you get breathless, stop for a while. You should aim to let the abdominal muscles move that lower hand at least three inches.

Sometimes it helps, if you are lying down, to put a tissue box on your abdomen so that you can see when you've made it move up and down with your breathing.

Some people imagine their lungs like a balloon. As you extend the abdominal muscles to allow air into the lower lungs, you are filling the base of your balloon. The air then fills the balloon of your middle and upper chest, bringing it into the throat area. When fully extended, your balloon is replenished with air, your chest cavity used as it is designed to be used.

The Out-breath

The out-breath is slower and is the most important part of the breathing cycle. It needs to take longer than the in-breath. At the end of the out-breath there is an almost vacuum state and we can pause in the suspension of this moment. I find it an almost magical aspect of the breathing cycle – the moment before the in-breath begins once again.

In the movement of the out-breath you will be releasing the used oxygen that has now passed all around your body and expelling carbon dioxide. Begin the letting-out process slowly and gently, first from the throat, then the middle area and then the diaphragm. You can aid the out-breath by actively pushing the air out very slowly, even making a growling noise to remind you of the process.

When we are stressed we frequently hyperventilate and use only the upper part of the chest, often tightening and raising the shoulders as we breathe. Many breathing problems occur because in an anxious state we focus on trying to gulp as much air in as possible, forgetting the important act of letting go. This process means that we take in too much oxygen and not enough carbon dioxide, so that the balance of the two is disturbed. The quick remedy for symptoms of hyperventilation – dizziness, cold hands and feet, anxiety – is to breathe in and out of a paper bag. This act restores the balance of oxygen and carbon dioxide to the body tissues, the lungs in particular.

2. *Mindfulness practice*

Breathing in, I have arrived. Breathing out, I am home.

THICH NHAT HANH, *The Miracle of Mindfulness*

Mindfulness is a means of awakening and maintaining your full attention in the present moment. This means that, instead of being pulled about by ideas of the past or the future, you are able to truly focus on what is, in the here and now. This helps you maintain an awareness of your feelings, your body, and thus your feeling and physical heart. Mindfulness practice brings you home to yourself and offers you liberation from the attachments that create suffering.

When we practise awareness of breathing we see that breathing affects our mind and our mind affects our body. Thus awareness of breathing is also awareness of the body.

In 'forgetfulness' you are pulled about by the mind that encompasses thoughts and emotions as you plot and plan your next move, fuelling potential disasters in your imagination, or going over and over the past and feeling dragged down by it. Thinking 'Why did he do that to me five years ago?' or 'It's not fair' or 'I blame my parents' or 'If I'd accepted that job in 1980 I would be OK now' makes the heart sore.

Liberation from forgetfulness via mindfulness does not mean avoiding feeling, but penetrating it, sometimes transforming it, in order to be fully awake.

We keep ourselves 'fresh' by the daily renewal practices. We may practise mindfulness of breathing, mindfulness of walking, mindfulness of eating, mindfulness of talking with another person.

● MINDFULNESS OF BREATHING

This practice is another way of sitting just with yourself and all your experiences and feelings and offering a loving kindness to yourself. This practice helps to distribute calmness to the whole body, in particular to the heart, and also helps you to be in touch with both your feeling heart and your physical heart.

● Find a place to sit comfortably with your back straight. If you are unwell you can also do this practice lying down. The concentration in this breathing exercise is simply on the nature of the breath itself. Find a place where you can concentrate upon imagining your breath entering your body. Choose just under the nostrils, or the throat, or the abdomen.

● Just breathe in, concentrating only on the breath.

● Then let the breath go by following it down on the out-breath, returning the breath that has been used by the body.

● Then, breathe in the fresh air to be taken up by the body once again, the air for your lungs, providing the oxygen for your heart.

● Continue with this cycle of gentle breathing, concentrating only on the breath itself.

● Every time a thought enters your mind, just note it, let it go and return to the breath. Thoughts will come. Don't try and prevent them or reject them, just note them. Do not water the seeds of thoughts by giving them energy.

You may notice that your breath actually has a quality about it. Some days it may feel light, or silky, or strong; sometimes harsh, limited, even sore. Just note this quality and return to the breath with your kindness and compassion.

Sit with just your breathing for about ten minutes at first, once a day. In time you might want to increase the time.

> It only needs one conscious breath to be back in contact with yourself, three conscious breaths to maintain that contact.

You can practise mindfulness of breathing at any time, wherever you are. The practice of mindfulness itself can be brought into every daily task – household tasks, work, travelling, looking after children, cooking, gardening, exercising all take on a more pleasant and joyful sense of presence when we do them mindfully, because we are concentrating upon the present moment and are not distracted by other thoughts. When we catch ourselves becoming 'forgetful', we can just say, 'Ah,' and return to the breath.

● MINDFULNESS OF FEELING

This exercise follows the same process as mindfulness of breathing except that the emphasis is upon feelings.

● Breathing in, you are aware of feeling.

● Breathing out, you are aware of feeling.

You may experience the feeling in your body. Your neck or back might ache, you might feel something in the pit of your stomach. You may feel sad, anxious, even angry. Whatever the form of feeling, give it your loving attention. Breathe it in and breathe it out. For example, once you have sensed that you are carrying anger, just breathe in the anger and then breathe out the anger. Often, just this simple process changes the experience of anger. It softens or dissolves.

Feelings themselves are quite simple – we feel glad, sad, happy, hurt, but we can make them into bigger structures like emotion. It is useful to notice every time this happens. In his book *Breath by Breath* Larry Rosenberg writes about how such practices help to reveal to us the constructs we all put around feelings that makes them into a much bigger deal. If we notice when this happens, we can release harmful emotions and heal our heart.

ALICE

Alice began mindfulness of feeling practice after struggling with high blood pressure. She noted, as she breathed in to her feelings in her chest, that they were feelings of hurt. As she breathed with the hurt, she noticed how her mind began coming in with all sorts of ideas about the hurt. 'You have every right to be hurt. They did awful things to you. Don't let them get away with it.' She could see that her feelings of hurt could quite quickly move into big emotions of anger and revenge and that these emotions could take on a rigid quality, hard to soften or shift. They had 'hardened down' into her heart, pushing up her blood pressure.

As she got used to the practice and simply returned to the feeling of being hurt, she could also feel sad. The sadness offered up tears and she found herself sobbing after one of the practices. This brought a spaciousness to both her heart-space and her feelings. There was movement and more space. She returned to the feelings to allow them to flow where they needed, simply breathing in to them and out with them, the breathing becoming like a river flowing over the stones and rocks of the events of her life.

Exercising Body and Soul

Once your fitness level is on an even keel and you have the go-ahead from the doctor, then a programme of daily exercise is essential for keeping mind, body and soul in harmony.

Before exercise of any kind you need to check out how your

body actually feels. This will be an individual matter and any exercise programme needs to be tailored to the individual. Also, your body may respond more strongly to stressors one day than the next.

Energy Bank Check

♦ Learn to sit with your body first thing in the morning and get a sense of how much energy there is in its energy bank. Just feel into your whole body by 'sweeping' its different areas, noting, as you go, how each part of you feels in terms of energy. Your legs may feel full of energy but your chest area may be saying 'Let me rest for a while.' Checking the energy bank helps you to discriminate in terms of the use of energy by selecting what is most important at that time and place.

♦ Then think about the activities you are proposing to do that day.

♦ Having gone through them, feel your body's reaction. Does it feel as if you will be using 50 per cent of your energy, or 75 per cent, or will you be demanding energy from your reserve tank by the end of the day?

Getting used to this way of considering your body and its energy, you will be able to feel whether your body is ready to be exercised or whether it needs to be rested first. Returning to the example of Norman Cousins, you will remember that after preparing for his second treadmill test he was actually able to produce a lot more effort through his controlled action than when he was being driven from behind (*see page 135*). When you are being driven, on the run from that imaginary tiger, pouring those fight or flight hormones into your system, you compromise your adrenals, your lungs and your heart.

The most important understanding is that your exercise programme needs to be based upon your personal capacity and all aspects of your being should be taken into account. Many people compromise their exercise programme by being too competitive and wanting to rush ahead rather than proceeding step by step. Your capacity for exercise needs to be evaluated on a daily basis, to take into consideration tiredness, preoccupation, lack of concentration and heart and lung function. Listening to your body and your feelings and attitude will help you to set realistic limits.

Exercise always increases pulse rate and blood pressure. Learn to take your own pulse so that you can monitor its acceleration. You can find your pulse in the wrist by pressing two fingers along the bone in alignment with the thumb, and also in your neck by moving down between the chin and the ear until you find the beat. It takes some practice and it's useful to learn from someone skilled in pulse taking.

You may also keep a blood pressure gauge in your home for monitoring blood pressure three or four times each week. Blood pressure readings should be taken over a period of time and not judged from a one-off reading. If, having become accustomed to taking your own blood pressure, you are concerned about high or low readings, go directly to your doctor.

The following are suggestions for beginning an exercise programme slowly:

♦ Start with warm-up exercises such as basic stretching learned from a physiotherapist to warm the muscles and stimulate the blood flow.

♦ Undertake gradual non-competitive exercise such as walking or swimming, so that you build your capacity for exercise slowly and according to the amount of effort in the energy bank. Walking every day is ideal.

♦ Try non-competitive golf, tennis or other sports as a way of keeping your body in touch with how it feels to exercise.

It is always helpful to work with a specialist exercise coach who understands about effort and the workings of the heart. You will need to discriminate between a coach who is trained to push you hard, as if preparing an athlete, and a coach who puts your heart function first and enables you to be aware of it and progress at your own pace.

Feeding Body and Soul

Lose Weight Now

In our industrialised, wealthy nations, we have a huge choice of food and yet it seems that we do not know how to eat in a healthy, happy way. Most of us consume too many calories and eat an unbalanced diet. Over a third of British women and a quarter of British men are seriously overweight. Being fat is linked with higher cholesterol and higher blood pressure and you may not be able to exercise or even move at a normal pace.

> The moderately overweight are 80 per cent more at risk of heart disease than leaner people.

If you are overweight and have a heart problem it makes sense to concentrate upon gradually trying to lose weight. Joining a slimming club or creating a buddy system losing weight group is really helpful and encouraging. Many people overeat because they are lonely, depressed and unmotivated. Joining forces with others can help create the motivation you need.

> Try to think of losing weight as a positive gain for your heart rather than a vile deprivation.

Eat Sensibly

There are many research studies into the effect of dietary changes in people who already have heart disease. The trials conducted in the United States by Dr Dean Ornish have been widely publicised. His very strict vegetarian diet recommends taking less than 10 per cent of calories from fat, significantly lower than the World Health Organisation's recommendation of a heart health maintenance diet of 30 per cent of calories from fat. While Dr Ornish's trials do seem to indicate that it is possible to at least halt the progression of atherosclerosis by following his recommendations, his programme (which includes yoga and visualisation exercises as well as diet) is intense and can be hard to follow. If this kind of rigour is for you, then go for it. If not, don't be bullied into taking on something that makes you miserable, that is soul destroying. Choose a healthy programme for feeding your body, with your soul in mind, which you are likely to really stick to and have success with.

There is plenty of research to show that eating raw foods helps prevent heart attacks and these foods can be eaten freely. One 17-year study showed that people eating fresh fruit every day are less likely to suffer heart problems, with 24 per cent less fatal heart disease. The same study revealed that if you have a raw salad every day your risk of fatal heart disease is lowered by 26 per cent.

Getting obsessional or faddish about diet, however, is not helpful. It can do more harm than good. We've always been impressed with an approach to food that is mindful and which utilises foods that are fresh, grown locally and are easily available. If you are not familiar with cooking fresh vegetables or making use of grains, you can easily learn about this through the variety of books available in supermarkets, programmes on television and local courses on offer. You may know someone who can teach you. Ask your friends how they cook rice and pasta and make grains tasty! In a city and on a low income finding and affording fresh ingredients can be difficult, but the principle of changing your diet to a more healthy one is worth striving for.

Ways of eating affect hunger. Eating 'on the run', standing up, driving a car, walking in the street or grabbing a burger or pizza to eat on the bus or tube is not good for your digestion, or for your eating habits generally. Often, eating in this way is simply not satisfying either. It's as if we've not been aware of actual eating, just of stuffing something in. We feel full, even bloated, and yet we are still hungry somewhere. Also, fast foods and convenience foods are notoriously high in salt, sugar and fat – which is why they are so appealing. But they create a craving for more!

Food which has been carefully prepared, which is shared, over which time is taken, is generally more satisfying and appeases our hunger. Also, if you can eat slowly and wait for 20 minutes for the food to be taken in properly by your system, you will find that you won't want more.

● MINDFULNESS OF EATING

- First select the food you are to eat. Choose something you really like and arrange it on a really attractive plate in an appealing way, so that it looks nice, so that it looks like something to celebrate.

- Sit down with the plate in front of you.

- Give a short bow to the food in recognition of all the processes it has gone through to reach you. For example, rice is first nourished by the rain and ripened by the sun, then it is gathered from the fields by human hands, carried by lorry, and packaged by more hands and cooked by others. All these processes are in each grain of rice we eat.

- Eat slowly, taking your time, chewing each mouthful carefully at least ten times. Your bowl of rice may take 15 or 20 minutes to eat, but you will be enjoying a real 'exchange' with your food as perhaps never before.

At the end of the meal, you will be satisfied and will not want more.

Vitamin Supplements

Most vitamin supplements have not been found to be of particular benefit in heart disease. Vitamin E does appear to have some beneficial effects at medium doses (12 iu per day). Supplements of 200 iu, which are found in many supermarkets, taken twice a week, may be sensible and have been recommended by the magazine *Health Now*. Don't exceed the dose in the belief that more is better; too much seems to have the reverse effect.

You may wish to consult a nutritional therapist to discuss your diet and use of vitamins and supplements. In the UK the National Health Service provides advice from dieticians only within hospital settings and they tend to concentrate upon medical health needs. Nutritional therapy in the private sector is becoming more popular in North America and Europe. Food allergy is also an area of study that is increasing in our culture as more and more people discover allergies to chemicals and preservatives in food. As for food supplements, there are many views about taking these. If you are drawn to undertake some research for yourself into these areas, find a good responsible person to talk to or a text and read up on them. It is important not to become faddy or fixed. Here's a dietary prescription:

Dietary Prescription for the 21st Century

♦ Plenty of fruits, vegetables and salads with moderate amounts of salad oils (15–20 ml of olive, flax or rapeseed oil) or nuts.

♦ Moderate amounts of fish and lean meat, milk and cheese and unrefined starchy foods (bread, pasta, rice), and small amounts of spreads containing stanols or sterols (20–25 g/day).

- Regular physical activity (at least 30 minutes of walking per day), preferably after meals as this reduces the amount of fats circulating in the bloodstream.

- An optional 1–2 glasses of wine (preferably red) per day, taken with meals.

- Possibly tea rather than coffee – tea contains flavonoids that have powerful anti-atherosclerotic properties.

- Vitamins C and E, which are antioxidants and help scavenge 'free radicals' that damage the linings of the arteries.

- Folic acid, which helps to lower levels of homocysteine, high levels of which appear to be a risk factor for heart disease.

Smoking, Alcohol and Recreational Drugs

Smoking

We have already outlined the effects upon the heart of cigarette smoking (*see pages 80–1*). Smoking is definitely dangerous for the heart, but it is never too late to stop. Here are some tips:

- Plan a date to stop.

- Stop suddenly and make yourself throw away the packet with cigarettes in it. Don't stop gradually, as that way you often don't succeed.

- List the reasons you want to stop, for example your health, your family's health, the money you would save, no smell in the house, on your clothes, or on your breath, fewer lines on your face, especially around your mouth.

- Practise how you will reply when someone offers you a cigarette after you have given up.

- Put aside the money you would have spent on cigarettes and plan how you will spend it after a month.

• Think about the times you know you will be tempted – after a meal or at a party, for example – and devise other things to do at those times.

• Stop completely – don't shift to cigars and pipes.

Smoking is a habit and an addiction to nicotine. To overcome the addiction, nicotine replacement therapy may be very useful, in the form of patches or chewing gum.

A new drug, Bupropion, has recently been licensed to stop people smoking. It appears very effective in the early trials and also reduces weight gain during the treatment period. The main side-effects are insomnia and a dry mouth.

Hypnosis can be helpful in giving up smoking, and sometimes patients have found acupuncture helpful. If smoking has become habitual as a way of relaxing, finding an alternative route to relaxation can also help the process of giving up. Massage, Alexander Technique, yoga and tai chi all relax the body and mind and may well help you to feel more in control of the cravings for nicotine.

Alcohol

There is a good body of evidence which shows that one or two drinks per day lowers the risk of heart disease and may also lower the risk of Alzheimer's disease. Not drinking at all is associated with an increased risk of heart disease and heavy drinking (more that five glasses a day) is associated with a threefold increase in risk.

Although any alcohol probably provides this beneficial effect, it does appear to be red wine which is the most beneficial. The tannins (white wine does not have much in the way of tannins) and alcohol each enhance the other's anti-thrombotic (anti-clotting) and antioxidant effects (antioxidants scavenge free radicals throughout the body, cleaning it up). In addition alcohol dilates the arteries and veins.

Beer and spirits intake needs to be watched, however. All

alcohol is high in calories and in large quantities will increase weight. Also, the effect of alcohol upon the liver and in making the body toxic is considerable, and this will make a demand upon the heart. Habitual excess alcohol leading to alcoholic behaviour is behind many personal tragedies, often perpetuating isolation and depressive cycles, as well as seriously compromising the heart.

Recreational Drugs

Cocaine, amphetamine and Ecstasy have adverse effects on the heart and circulation, mainly by activating the sympathetic nervous system and increasing levels of adrenaline/noradrenaline. This leads to an increase in heart rate, constriction of arteries in the body, unpredictable blood pressure effects and heart rhythm disturbances. Habitual use of amphetamine and cocaine can cause repetitive episodes of spasm of the coronary arteries and paroxysms of high blood pressure. This may lead to heart attacks, angina and possibly dilated flabby hearts (dilated cardiomyopathy).

Cocaine can in some instances lead to marked slowing of the heart or complete heart block. A February 2001 *British Medical Journal* article revealed a study that showed that one-quarter of non-fatal heart attacks in the United States were in users of cocaine. Also, cocaine is estimated to increase the risk of heart attack by 58 per cent.

Cannabis has a biphasic effect. At low/moderate doses it produces an increase in heart rate and cardiac output, whereas at high doses it produces a slowing of the heart rate and low blood pressure. There is also an increase in ectopic beats (both ventricular and supraventricular). In people with coronary heart disease, cannabis increases the frequency of anginal symptoms at low levels of exercise.

Connecting Body and Soul

Looking after your heart can involve many different practices and take you into areas you may never have imagined. Remember, whatever is nourishing for your heart on the levels of body, mind, feeling and spirit will help the healing and well-being of your heart.

At times of great demand, when the pain in your chest reminds you of your vulnerability, it is helpful to be able to stop and meet these times calmly and thus feel less at their mercy.

The mindfulness practices are a way of being very still with your body, mind and emotions. The stillness will help you appreciate what your body and psyche are carrying. Feelings such as fear, anxiety and rage, which have been either repressed or denied for years due to ignorance, can be recognised and softened, releasing their toxicity from the heartspace.

Regular practice of mindfulness keeps us in touch with ourselves, with the still, small point or voice within, with our spirit.

MARK

Mark's father died from a heart attack and then his baby daughter Esther came close to death because of a serious heart infection in the same year. Mark remembers sitting in Southwark cathedral waiting for the ambulance to arrive from Brighton with his family – his wife Rachel, eight-month-old Esther and one-year-old Laurie:

> Esther had been not breathing well, her temperature had rocketed up and her body wasn't coping. The doctor had said, 'It looks as if she's got an enormous heart, but it can't be true.' I was thinking, 'What if she has, what if she has a big heart?'

At Guy's, the ultrasound proved her heart was enlarged with fluid around it.

> She was in this mass of wires and tubes, lying there, alert in her eyes, but physically not moving much. Her heart was infected with masses of fluid.

Mark found that Esther's illness offered him an opportunity to become more intimate with his father and his memory. Mark's father had had angina and a heart attack when Mark was in his early twenties.

> He never had any sense of what his heart meant. I feel a sort of loving compassionate anger about that. If he had had a sense of connectedness to his own heart or his own body, which I feel I have, he could have lived a bit longer. When he did die of a heart attack at 76 it was very sudden.
>
> I think what would have helped me with my dad and with Esther would have been having information in a way that gave me a picture of what the illness was. I find visualisation really helpful. My image of my own heart is of it being slightly shrivelled and shrunken and I am alarmed by that. I realise that as well as taking care of my body, I must also take care of my emotions. The heart is nourished through intimacy, through being in tune somehow with my sense of self, my will and spirit, in a way that I don't think my dad knew.... Part of my search now is trying to keep a spiritual connection with my dad and it's as if I want this because I don't want to lose intimacy, I need to keep it going in order to nurture my own heart. My dad would be pleased to know that through his death has come a deeper understanding of the experience of spirit and of death.

Visualisation and Relaxation

These exercises are two important self-help tools you can use at any time, anywhere. Visualisation involves using our imagination and thus is a more 'active' mental process where we go somewhere in our minds, or enter the chambers of our heart. Relaxation involves us in the process of using our minds to relax our muscles and let go of thoughts, slowing our breathing and heart rate, to give the whole body a complete rest. We are always stunned at the impact of people's imaginative efforts on their bodies. We recently heard an incredibly moving account of a political prisoner in solitary confinement who was helped to survive his terrible ordeal by deciding each day where he would go – a day trip to Paris, a ride on a gondola in Venice, a walk in the Rocky Mountains. He was helped by sharing these plans with other prisoners in solitary who could shout to each other through the wall, taking each other on a detailed imaginative journey.

Visualisation can also have a powerful healing effect on the body itself and has been well researched by Carl and Stephanie Simonton in cancer patients who were invited to imagine the cancer cells inside their body and what should happen to them so that they did not compromise the entire body. Some people imagined them being swept into a deep pool and being cleansed; others imagined a line of soldiers crunching them up. One young boy imagined his pancreas as a factory manufacturing insulin to balance the sugar in red blood cells. His body needed the production to increase and so the boy imagined extra help!

Such exercises are useful in the management and experience of suffering in the body. They always have a beneficial effect upon the person as a whole and often have an effect upon the disease process itself.

You may find visualisation or relaxation tapes in bookstores or health shops. You might like to make a tape of your own using the voice of someone you love, your favourite music, birdsong or ocean waves. Visualisation exercises involve your own unique imagination and your inner world. After closing your eyes and relaxing, you allow your imagination to respond to the guided conversation and requests. It is important to allow images or feelings to emerge, whatever they may be. Do not try to judge them or control them, but let your own self respond. There is no 'right' response. It is simply important for your own language to be allowed to flow, like a river, so that you are connecting deeply with your own inner world and metaphors.

The yoga and relaxation teacher Moira MacLean, who died a few months ago, came to talk to me (Elizabeth) and offered the following contribution to this book. She worked with patients for many years, offering meditations for healing and deep relaxation, taking mindfulness into the body. She had serene commitment to the process of dying and spent her professional life helping others to be in touch with the energy she calls 'heart energy': 'When words are no longer adequate, you can send love from your heart to the heart of another.'

Moira also used heart meditation for being present with her husband, who had Alzheimer's disease and was often confused and disorientated. She felt we are all responsible for the energies we transmit into the world and to others.

Here is the visualisation exercise Moira gave to her patients. Find someone who will read the exercise to you as you lie down in a comfortable place and relax.

● INNER LOVE VISUALISATION

Become aware of your heart, right in the middle of the chest. Make sure your mouth remains closed and imagine you are breathing in and out through the heart centre. Try and make your breathing rhythmic and be completely aware of each incoming and outgoing breath. Allow several minutes to pass to deepen awareness.

Now imagine the air you are breathing in is of a golden colour – it is like a golden mist – and you are taking this golden mist into your heart. Feel it radiating out of your heart and filling your body, down into the trunk, into your legs and feet, up into your chest, down your arms into your hands, up into your neck and into your head. Your whole body is filled with this golden mist. Feel that every time you breathe in you are cleaning out your whole body and the golden mist is giving you many good qualities – love, peace, compassion, serenity, acceptance, openness and honesty.

Breathe out all the things you don't want or like about yourself – fear, anger, confusion, criticism, resentment. . . . All these things are carried away by the golden mist.

Now become aware of your heartbeat. Listen to the steady sound of your heart and imagine that the golden mist has formed into a very small, golden egg in your heart. As you watch, the golden egg breaks open, and there in your heart, sitting on a beautiful flower, is a tiny little being. This little being is surrounded by a cloud of bright light. It is sitting very still and silently looking at you, sending you wave upon wave of pure love and peace. Let yourself be filled with this love – all you have to do is receive. This little being is sending you so much love and the more it gives, the brighter it becomes. It is giving you so much that you cannot keep it all inside you. Think of the people you love, family, friends, the sick, lonely, unhappy people in the world, and send them this love. Think of the people you don't like – send them love. The more love you send out, the more the little being in your chest fills you with love.

Now it is time to leave the little being. Very gently the petals close and the egg becomes whole again ... but remember, the little being always remains in your heart, you only have to look for it.

A colleague Susie Nixon offers the next visualisation exercise to her heart patients and to this book. Again, find a comfortable place to sit or lie and invite a friend to read you the following:

● THE HOUSE OF THE HEART VISUALISATION

Find yourself standing in a field, with the sun overhead. It is summer. Notice the atmosphere, landscape and feeling of the field – its sights, sounds, smells.

Near the field is a house. This is your house. Notice what it is made of, how it looks.

When you are ready, enter the house. Walk into the hall and notice the number of rooms.

In one room you will hear a rhythmic pounding and you will know that this is the room representing your own heart. As you enter this room, take a good look round. If there is anything in the room that seems out of sorts, disconnected, dark or unhealthy, go towards this part of the room and place your own healing hands upon it. As you are doing this, ask:

'What does my heart need most?'
'What is it that I'm not doing that my heart needs?'
'If you could speak, heart, what would you say?'

As you stay with whatever emerges in this exercise, become aware of your own capacity for healing and for holding the wisdom of your own heart. Believe in this natural wisdom and knowing.

Working with Dreams

Dreams are seen by therapists as the 'royal road' to unconscious processes. Dreams help us to become aware of energies that remain hidden from us during the day when we are mostly preoccupied with conscious matters. Dreams have an important part to play in the balance of our psychological and emotional life.

Dreams are simple messages in code; they are often larger than life in order for us to take notice of their messages. They may speak of hidden aspects of ourselves; they may draw our attention to what remains in the shadow of our being; they may offer us images of healing; they may be moving and transformative. People who become familiar with the language of their dreams find the information gathered helpful. Dreams sometimes contain answers to daily puzzles and problems. Rather than trying to interpret a dream, let its energy, feeling and images find a place within you. Writing your dreams down helps to give them a valid part in your everyday world.

If you don't remember your dreams, but want to know about your unconscious life, try asking for a dream that would indicate how things are inside your unconscious mind. You might also try asking for a dream about your heart and see what that brings forth.

Chapter 17

COMPLEMENTARY THERAPIES FOR THE HEART

Complementary medicine is increasingly practised in conventional medical settings, particularly acupuncture for pain, and massage, music therapy, and relaxation techniques for mild anxiety and depression.

A clinical review of complementary medicine in the *British Medical Journal*, September 2000

THERE ARE MANY kinds of professional support for your problems with your heart. They range from the psychological, via psychotherapy and counselling, through complementary medicine, such as acupuncture, homoeopathy and Chinese herbalism, to practices such as massage, yoga, Alexander Technique, mindfulness practice, prayer and meditation. Complementary therapies may include both touch and an invitation for you to use your imagination, as in visualisation.

These therapies are for your own 'self-help' in support of the medical services you may be receiving. *They are not an alternative to the treatment you have been receiving.*

Medical Services

It is very important to feel secure in the approach of your medical services towards helping you with your heart. Some people feel nervous about asking questions of their medical services. But if you feel that your questions have not been answered fully, or you have concerns about your treatment, you are allowed to seek a second opinion. Get support for this decision from friends or from consulting another professional in an allied area. It may be that, having read some of the information in this book, you have a clearer understanding of what areas of concern you would like your current medical services to address.

Every area throughout the world is different. What is available locally will vary tremendously. Some areas, such as the west of England, the west coast of the United States, Germany and the south of France, are rich in complementary medicine and have a growing demand for complementary approaches. Some private health insurance companies now include a contribution towards homoeopathy, acupuncture and osteopathy, and this will be worth investigation. Private practitioners will all charge a fee, and this may be costly. Many practitioners work on a sliding scale according to your financial position. The growing number of health centres in Britain, other parts of Europe and the United States and Canada where complementary medicine is offered attest to the interest in this field.

As you read through this chapter, just 'tune in' to the kinds of therapy that might be useful to you in terms of what you need for both your feeling and your physical heart.

Support from Professionals

The choice of individual therapist is very important, as is their theoretic orientation. You need to feel a rapport in order to work in a therapeutic alliance.

Psychotherapy and Counselling

The main difference between psychotherapy and counselling is that, very broadly speaking, psychotherapy works at a greater depth and for longer than counselling. Both are effective forms of intervention for emotional stress that is hard to reach with your own self-help exercises. The theoretical approach of the psychology mentioned throughout this book comes from Cognitive Analytic Therapy and Transpersonal Psychology (*see Resources, page 251*).

If you decide to seek the help of a psychological therapist, do a bit of research first. You may go through your doctor; in fact many practices have resident professionals several days a week. You may write to the British Association for Counsellors or the United Kingdom Council for Psychotherapy to ask for an accredited therapist in your area (*see Resources, page 251*).

Holistic Practitioners

A holistic practitioner looks at the whole person. At your initial consultation you will be asked about your likes and dislikes, your tastes and habits, your feelings, dreams and disappointments and your personal and family history as well as your symptoms. Choose a practitioner who is qualified and accredited, especially if they have been personally recommended to you.

Acupuncture

Acupuncture is a traditional Chinese procedure involving the insertion of needles along meridians in the body. Research findings show that acupuncture has a pain-relieving effect and helps 70 per cent of patients with angina.

In *Healing the Heart* Chinese acupuncturist and herbalist Man Xing Chowkwanyun writes:

In Chinese medicine The Heart (HE) ranks as sovereign in the hierarchy of organs. On the physical level the HE maintains the circulation of blood, the ability to speak, the perception of taste, consciousness, clarity of thinking, memory and the ability to sleep. On the feeling level the HE maintains the ability to love, *joie de vivre*, inspiration, creativity, self-esteem and the ability to dream. Chinese medicine contributes both to the prevention and healing of HE disorders.

Alexander Technique

Change involves carrying out an activity against the habits of a lifetime.

F. M. ALEXANDER

The Alexander Technique was developed a century ago by an Australian actor who had lost his voice while reciting Shakespeare. Through self-observation he noticed that his habit of pulling his head back and down while speaking was the cause of his vocal problems. By correcting the relationship of neck, head and spine, his speech returned. In the 1930s he began training people in London to conduct the Alexander Technique to bring about postural changes.

The technique's efficacy has been acknowledged in studies reported in the *Lancet* and the *British Medical Journal*. It is entirely safe and produces a harmonious effect on both mind and body and helps a number of conditions, ranging from back pain to headaches. The technique releases a sense of balance and freedom from the stresses upon the body caused by poor posture and can be a great help with poor breathing habits, which are often implicated in heart disease.

There are trained Alexander Technique teachers all over the world who will offer individual courses of treatment so that the technique can become part of everyday life.

Biofeedback

Biofeedback instruments were developed to help people observe the changes in their body temperature, pulse and brain-waves in response to relaxation, visualisation and meditation techniques. The instruments do not affect the body in any way – they just provide information. Biofeedback training affects the autonomic nervous system, which governs responses such as blood pressure, skin temperature, digestion and muscular tension. Hyperventilation and panic attacks may be controlled by learning breathing techniques with the aid of biofeedback.

Some doctors have biofeedback machines in their practices and staff to offer training to patients. Biofeedback machines are also available for use at home for people to teach themselves to relax.

Cranial Osteopathy

A cranial osteopath is a qualified osteopath who has specialised in working with the eight bones of the cranium and the nerves that originate in the brain that affect different parts of the body. This work is extremely subtle and is known to help conditions such as high blood pressure and circulation and breathing problems, as well as migraine and stomach ulcers. Many cranial osteopaths also work with the subtle energy bodies of the individual and thus their work includes degrees of hands-on healing. Their approach is similar to that of Chinese medicine in terms of treating the whole person and their body/mind system.

Some cranial osteopaths work in health clinics, but most are in private practice.

Homoeopathy

This system of healing is based upon the natural law of 'like cures like'. The foundations of classical homoeopathy were laid down by Samuel Hahnemann (1755–1843).

Homoeopathy treats the whole person and a practising homoeopath will encourage the patient to tell their story in their own way, including their hopes and fears as well as their reactions to environment, weather, stress, food, people and work.

Two good trials have established that homoeopathy is effective in the prevention and treatment of heart disease. One trial revealed that 75 per cent of patients showed improvement in their blood pressure readings and were able to reduce their drug treatment. Any homoeopathic medicine must be prescribed by a qualified homoeopath who has taken your history. The exception to this is Arnica 6, which is very good for shock and is available in most chemists.

Aromatherapy, Massage and Reflexology

All three of these therapies involve touch, the laying on of hands. Touch itself is one of the most important aspects of all approaches to healing. James Lynch, in *The Broken Heart*, writes: 'For unconscious arrhythmic heart patients, manual pulse taking had a normalising effect on the heart rhythm.'

Aromatherapy

Complementary medicine consultant Dr Jane Buckle has lectured extensively throughout Britain and the United States on the invaluable potency of touch for all levels of healing – body, mind and emotions. She teaches nurses as well as other health professionals a technique called the M-technique, which combines gentle touch with essential oils. She states that aromatherapy can be used in situations where massage cannot – for example when someone is very fragile following surgery or when a person's circulation is compromised. As she is also a specialist in aromatherapy, she has made a detailed study of the effect of both the inhalation of aromatic oils and their application through the skin. The anxiety level of a hospital admission may respond to the calming effects of lavender (*Lavandula augustifolia*) or Roman chamomile (*Anthemis nobilis*).

Essential oils can be used for relaxation, to promote sleep, to soothe the pain of arthritis and to prevent cross-infection. Some oils should be avoided by heart patients, such as rosemary and spike lavender, which are stimulant. Essential oil of rose (*Rosa damascena*) is particularly soothing for recovery from surgery and heart attack.

The power of smell to evoke memory is well known. Dr Buckle suggests using both fragrances from oils, which carry a harmonious pleasurable memory, and the gentle kindness of touch during periods of hospitalisation and recovery at home.

Oils may be used in a burner, putting just a few drops into water which is heated by a candle underneath. Two or three drops of essential oil (the pure kind, not an amalgam) can be added to a base oil such as almond oil for the use of massage at home. Just massaging feet makes a difference. Many hospitals will support relatives massaging the feet of their loved one.

Massage
Massage aids the release of endorphins, some of which, enkephalins, are known to be as powerful as morphine. Massage also aids the lymphatic system, allowing the body to release fluid and toxins from stress and poor diet.

Studies have shown that massage, with its hands-on touch from a dedicated massage therapist, can lower the pulse rate and blood pressure as well as helping patients to feel connected to their own system of self-healing.

Reflexology
Reflexology involves pressing points on the soles of the feet that correspond to different organs within the body. The central part of the sole next to the ball of the foot reflects the heart.

Heart surgeon Mehmet Oz writes in *Healing from the Heart* that he began to spontaneously massage the feet of a patient in whom he had just inserted a LVAD artificial heart pump and whose heart had begun to fail. With nothing else available to help his patient, Dr Oz kept up the foot massage for 45 minutes until the monitor registering the blood flow across his patient's lungs showed a steady improvement.

Healing Hands

There are undoubtedly some extremely gifted healers working in all settings. Many medical practitioners also have natural healing qualities or healing hands.

A healer will ask you to sit or lie and, in silence, will use their hands at just a short distance over your body to conduct healing energy. A skilled healer will be able to locate, through their hands, the area of suffering in your body and feelings. Their work will be more effective if you are able to surrender to the process, for the gift of healing comes through the meeting of two individuals and two souls.

Most healers ask for donations in exchange for the work they do rather than a fixed fee. Many people I know have received enormous help from their visits to healers, both in terms of the connection they have felt to an energy force within themselves, and a calming and encouraging sense that such exchange of energy is possible.

The gifted healer Allegra Taylor's book *I Fly Out with Bright Feathers* is an inspiration to anyone interested in developing their own healing potential, as well as containing fascinating information about healing traditions and healers all over the world.

Spiritual Healing and Prayer

Surveys in America have shown that of all the non-medical healing practices, prayer is the most common. A study into absent healing at the University of California Medical School found that patients who were prayed for needed fewer antibiotics and were less likely to develop heart failure.

People who have a strong religious faith or who follow a spiritual tradition do seem to have that protective skin of 'hardiness'. Not only is spiritual practice and prayer helpful for the spirit, but it is also good for your heart! Also, at times of difficulty, during surgery, intensive care and especially during the process of dying, prayer is of great support both to the patient and their relatives.

TAKING RESPONSIBILITY FOR YOUR GIFT OF LIFE

And so I have travelled.
And the breath of all my ancestors is in this world,
And the breath of all my enemies,
The breath of the lame and the ignorant
and the breath of alienation and pain,
All goes through me;
And my gasps of pain and sobs of loss
Go out also, not to the void,
But to feed the earth,
Whence the tide turns to me tenfold
More than I give.

From 'Breath' by MARK DUNN, *Strange Days and Other Poems* (private collection)

WHETHER OR NOT you have suffered an emergency, the crisis of a new diagnosis, a heart attack or surgery, there is a great deal you can do to help your heart and a first important step is to take responsibility for this. Doctors can do a great deal for the heart and then it is up to you. When you are in a crisis or time of high stress, you may say, 'I will never get into this situation again.' Then, months later, when you feel better, it's all too easy to forget your positive resolutions. Old habits do take time to change.

However, there are many small steps that you can take in

daily life to support the function of your heart and to keep your emotional and spiritual heart open to the beauty of life.

A Peace Treaty with the Heart

The Zen Master Thich Nhat Hanh speaks about the possibility of peace in every step and peace in every cell of our body. He teaches the practice of mindful breathing where the practice itself becomes the bridge that links mind and body together. Upon this bridge we meet the very contents of our mind and mind's effect upon the body. Thus we nourish our 'telephone line' to the heart and bring peace to our body so that its capacity for self-healing is encouraged and enhanced.

● BREATHING EXERCISE

One of the most effective ways to bring peace into your heart is through the simple practice of breathing. Stop whatever it is you are doing now and try this simple exercise, with your eyes open or closed:

● Breathing in, become aware of your heart.

● Breathing out, smile to your heart.

● Breathing in, become aware of your heart.

● Breathing out, smile to your heart.

Repeat this exercise throughout the day. It will bring you a sense of peacefulness as well as maintaining the telephone link to your feeling heart. Whenever you stop and breathe alongside these words you will be looking after your physical and feeling heart. If there is anything stored in your heartspace, this exercise will reveal it so that you may take other steps to look after it, and the verses themselves will be nourishing.

APPENDIX

How to Recognise a Heart Attack and What to Do

The symptoms of a heart attack are severe crushing chest pain – it feels as though someone is sitting on your chest – nausea, breathlessness and sweating. You may look grey or pale. If this happens to you:

- Don't delay, thinking it is indigestion and may pass – take action.

- Ring for an ambulance.

- Chew a 300 mg aspirin (it will make the blood less sticky).

If you are present when someone has a heart attack and collapses, remember the ABC of resuscitation:

A is for Airway
Make sure that the mouth and airway are clear by putting a finger in the back of the throat. Sometimes the tongue can obstruct the airway, or dentures or vomit can cause a problem.

B is for Breathing
Check for breathing. If there are no signs, breathe into the person's mouth, and with your fingers pinching their nose blow a sufficient volume of air into their mouth – enough to make the chest rise and fall five times. You will give life-saving oxygen to the tissues, especially the brain.

C is for Circulation

Check for a pulse, either at the wrist or in the neck. Feel along the thick muscle which runs from the angle of the jaw to the collar-bone. Halfway down (on the side nearest the Adam's apple) is the carotid pulse.

If there is no pulse, then a simple thump on the chest may convert the very irregular heart beat of ventricular fibrillation into regular beating. Then, with the palm of one hand on the bottom of the chest bone (sternum) and the palm of the other hand on top, press down moderately (you are not aiming to break any ribs) 15 times in quick succession.

Then breathe again into the mouth as above and intersperse two breaths with 15 chest compressions. This is very tiring and you should get others to help and take over from you until assistance arrives.

Recovery Position

If the person recovers, turn them on their side with the arms positioned as shown below. The underneath leg should be straight and the other leg should be bent across it.

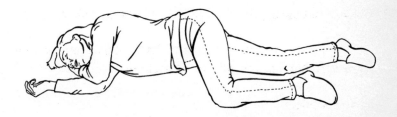

GLOSSARY

ACE inhibitor A type of drug that may be used for heart failure or high blood pressure. ACE stands for 'angiotensin converting enzyme' and works by blocking the formation of angiotensin, which narrows blood vessels.

Aneurysm A weak area in the wall of an artery or in the wall of the heart that can be pushed out in a mushroom-like effect.

Angina The feeling of pressure in the chest, sometimes described as 'like a vice'. It is dull, not sharp. The pain can radiate into the jaw, neck, arm and shoulders.

Angiocardiography An X-ray examination of the heart and coronary arteries. A catheter is inserted from the arm or leg and a dye that shows up on the X-ray machine is injected to show the arteries or the heart.

Angioplasty The technique whereby a catheter containing an inflatable balloon is inserted into a coronary artery. The balloon is inflated and the narrowing artery enlarged.

Anti-coagulant A drug such as heparin, Warfarin or tinnazaparin that increases the time taken for the blood to clot, thus making it thinner.

Aorta The main artery leading from the heart to the rest of the body.

Aortic valve The 'no-return' valve from the left ventricle (pump) to the aorta.

Arrhythmia An abnormal heart rhythm.

Artery A blood vessel carrying oxygenated blood to the tissues.

Atheroma A process whereby the inner layer of the arteries becomes thickened and fatty deposits are laid down.

Atrial fibrillation An irregular beating of the heart.

Atrium A receiving chamber of the heart. There are two – one on the right to receive venous (blue) blood and one on the left to receive arterial (red) blood with oxygen from the lungs.

Beta blocker A drug often given for angina and high blood pressure and increasingly for heart failure. It slows the heart down.

Blood pressure The pressure generated by the heart pump (ventricle) to push blood around the body.

Blue babies Babies who are born with a connection between the right (blue) side of the heart and the left (red) side of the heart, so that blue (venous) blood is mixed with the red (oxygenated) side of the circulation.

Bradycardia Slow heart rate.

CABG Coronary artery bypass grafting, sometimes called 'CABbaGe'. A surgical technique whereby a vein or an artery is taken from the aorta to beyond a narrowing in a coronary artery.

Calcium channel blocking agents Drugs often given for angina or high blood pressure.

Capillaries The very fine blood vessels that spread through organs. Small arteries supply oxygen-carrying red blood to capillaries and small veins take blue blood away from capillaries.

Cardiac arrest When the heart stops beating and there is no effective pumping.

Cardiomyopathy An abnormal muscle in the heart, either thickened or thinned. Either way it does not function normally.

Cardiopulmonary resuscitation (CPR) The technique used to try and make the heart and lungs work again when they have stopped.

Cardiovascular Relating to the heart and circulation.

Catheterisation A technique whereby a tube called a catheter is introduced into a vein or an artery and passed to the heart. Dye is then injected through the tube and areas of the heart, including the coronary arteries, which can be seen on the X-ray machine. The technique can also be used to measure pressure in the heart.

Cerebral thrombosis *See* Stroke.

Cerebrovascular accident (CVA) *See* Stroke.

Cholesterol A necessary fat found in the blood. Cholesterol is made up of two main parts: HDL, or high density lipoprotein, which is protective in heart disease, and LDL, or low density lipoprotein, which is harmful in heart disease.

Collateral circulation When there is a narrowing or a blockage in a main artery small channels can be opened up around the blockage to achieve flow further down the system.

Congenital defects Defects that are present from birth.

Coronary arteries Arteries that supply the heart muscle.

Coronary artery disease *See* Ischaemic heart disease.

Coronary or Cardiac Care Unit (CCU) A specialised unit for monitoring and treating patients immediately after a heart attack or patients with unstable angina.

Coronary thrombosis *See* Heart attack.

Cyanosis Blueness of the skin and lips, usually due to too little oxygen reaching the tissues.

Defibrillator A machine that gives an electric shock to the heart to try and restore regular beating.

Diabetes (Mellitus) A disease in which there is too much sugar in the blood caused by a lack of or resistance to insulin.

Diastolic pressure The resting pressure in the system after the heart has pumped.

Digoxin A tablet to help slow the heart rate. Sometimes given for heart failure.

Diuretic A drug that stimulates the kidneys to produce more urine.

Doppler ultrasound An ultrasound technique usually performed at the time of an echocardiogram to measure flow in the heart and blood vessels.

Echocardiogram A technique whereby a probe is placed on the chest wall and sound waves are directed towards the heart. These are reflected from different parts of the heart and are used to build up a picture of the structure of the heart and its function.

Electrocardiogram A recording of the electrical activity of the heart.

Embolus A clot of blood that starts in one part of the system and ends up elsewhere.

Endocarditis Infection of the heart valves or wall of the heart.

Exercise test A graduated walking test performed while attached to an electrocardiogram in order to assess the response of the heart to exercise.

Fibrillation An irregular and incoordinate contraction of the heart. This can just be the atria (receiving chambers of the heart), as in atrial fibrillation, when the heart can still beat adequately. Alternatively, it can be the ventricles – ventricular fibrillation, when no useful heart pumping action occurs and death follows.

Haemorrhage Bleeding.

Heart attack Blockage of a coronary artery leading to the death of part of the heart muscle. Also called myocardial infarction or coronary thrombosis.

Heart failure A general term used when a heart is simply not pumping as well as it should.

Heart murmur A noise heard in the heart in addition to the opening (lub) and closing (dup) of the heart valves.

High blood pressure (hypertension) Blood pressure found to be above 145/95 on a number of occasions is considered to be elevated.

Hypercholesterolaemia Too much cholesterol in the blood.

Hyperlipidaemia Too much fat in the blood (both cholesterol and triglyceride).

Hypertension *See* High blood pressure.

Hypoxia Not enough oxygen.

Incompetence Also known as regurgitation; when applied to a heart valve means that the valve is leaking.

Ischaemia Inadequate blood supply.

Ischaemic heart disease Heart disease caused by too little blood getting to the heart muscle through the coronary arteries. Also called coronary artery disease.

Lipid Another term for blood fat.

Marfan syndrome A disorder of the connective tissue of the body, usually found in tall thin people with very long arms who are double-jointed and sometimes have eye problems. May affect the aorta, aortic valve or mitral valve. Inherited in many cases.

Mitral valve The 'no-return' valve between the left atrium (left receiving chamber) and the left ventricle (pump).

Myocardial infarction *See* Heart attack.

Myocardium Heart muscle.

Oedema Swelling of part of the body due to accumulation of fluid in the tissues.

Pacemaker An electrical system inserted to make the heart beat at a normal rate when it has been very slow or sometimes very fast.

Palpitations An uncomfortable awareness of the heartbeat.

Pericardium A membrane that surrounds the heart muscle.

Platelet A small particle in the blood that is involved in the blood-clotting process.

Prophylaxis Prevention.

Prothesis An artificial tissue used in place of a heart valve.

Pulmonary Relating to the lungs.

Radioisotope A substance emitting a tiny and safe dose of radioactivity which can be measured with a camera when administered to document the function of an organ in the body.

Regurgitation *See* Incompetence.

Resuscitation An attempt to re-establish normal function of the heart and lungs.

Risk factor A factor known to be associated with an increased risk of heart disease.

Sphygmomanometer The machine used by doctors and nurses to measure the blood pressure.

Stenosis Narrowing, as in a valve which doesn't fully open.

Stethoscope An instrument used to listen to sounds within the body.

Syncope Sudden loss of consciousness.

Stroke Also known as cerebral thrombosis or cerebrovascular accident (CVA). Damage to the brain caused either by a clot in an artery leading to the brain or by bleeding (haemorrhage).

Systolic blood pressure The surge of pressure created by the heart pump to push blood around the body to send oxygen to the tissues.

Tachycardia Fast heart rate.

Thrombolysis A technique to dissolve a clot.

Thrombosis Blood clot inside a blood vessel or within the heart.

Vascular Relating to the blood vessels.

Vein A vessel carrying blood back to the heart.

Ventricular fibrillation An irregular and incoordinate contraction of the ventricles (pumps) which if not corrected quickly leads to death.

FURTHER READING

Jeanne Achterbery, *Imagery in Healing*, New Science Library, 1985
Robert Bly, *Iron John*, Rider, 1990
Jane Buckle, *Clinical Aromatherapy for Nurses*, Arnold, 1997
Pema Chodron, *When Things Fall Apart: Heart Advice for Difficult Times*, Shambhala, 1997
Norman Cousins, *Anatomy of an Illness*, New England Journal of Medicine, 1976
—, *The Healing Heart*, Norton, 1983
Germaine Greer, *The Change*, Hamish Hamilton, 1991
Jack Kornfield, *A Path with Heart*, Bantam, 1993
—, *After the Ecstasy, the Laundry*, Bantam, 2000
C. S. Lewis, *A Grief Observed*, Faber and Faber, 1961
James Lynch, *The Broken Heart: The Medical Consequences of Loneliness*, Harper & Row, 1979
Elizabeth Wilde McCormick, *Healing the Heart*, Optima, 1992
—, *Change for the Better*, Cassell, 1997
Caroline Myss, *Why People Don't Heal and How They Can*, Harmony Books, 1997
Dean Ornish, *Reversing Heart Disease*, Ballantine Books, 1990
—, *Love and Survival*, HarperCollins, 1998
Mehmet Oz, *Healing from the Heart*, Dutton, 1998
Paul Pearsall, *The Heart's Code: The True Stories of Organ Transplant Patients*, Thorsons, 1998
Candace Pert, *Molecules of Emotion*, Simon and Schuster, 1999
Larry Rosenberg, *Breath by Breath*, Thorsons, 2000
Carl and Stephanie Simonton, *Getting Well Again*, Bantam, 1978
Stephen T. Sinatra, *Heartbreak and Heart Disease*, Keats, 1996
Felicity Smart and Dr Diana Holdright, *Heart Health for Women*, Thorsons, 1995
Allegra Taylor, *Acquainted with the Night*, Fontana, 1985
—, *I Fly Out with Bright Feathers*, Fontana, 1987
Thich Nhat Hanh, *The Miracle of Mindfulness*, Vermilion
—, *The Sun, my Heart*, Vermillion, 1986
—, *Anger: Wisdom for Cooling the Flames*, Riverhead Books, 2001
John Welwood, *Journey of the Heart: Intimate Relationships and the Path of Love*, HarperCollins, 1990
David White, *Poems of Self-Compassion*

RESOURCES

Useful Addresses

ASH (Action on Smoking and Health)
109 Gloucester Place, London W1H 3PH
Tel: 0207 935 3519

The Association of Cognitive Analytic Therapists
Academic Psychiatry, Third Floor, South Wing, St Thomas's Hospital
London SE1 7EH
Tel: 0207 928 9292 ext 3769   Website: www.acat.org.uk

The Blood Pressure Association
Tel: 0208 725 0650

The British Association for Counselling and Psychotherapy
1 Regent Place, Rugby, Warwickshire CV21 2PJ
Tel: 0870 443 5252   Fax: 0870 443 5160

The British Cardiac Association
Tel: 020 7383 3887

The British Heart Foundation
14 Fitzhardinge Street, London W1H 4DH
Tel: 0207 935 0185   Website: www.bhf.org.uk

The Centre for Transpersonal Psychology
86a Marylebone High Street, London W1M 3DE
Tel: 0207 935 7350   Fax: 0207 935 2672

Cica Care
A self-adhesive gel sheet which can be very helpful for healing post-
operative scar tissue. In the UK it is expensive – about £36.50 for a

12 × 6 cm sheet – but it may even work for scars more than 20 years old.
Helpline: 01882 773508

Coronary Prevention Group
Plantation House, Suite 5/4 D&M, 31/35 Fenchurch Street,
London EC3M 3NN
Tel: 0207 626 4844

Down's Heart Group
48 Main Street, Lyddington, Rutland LE15 9LT
Tel: 01572 822417

The Down's Syndrome Association
155 Mitcham Road, London SW17 7PG
Tel: 0208 682 4001

The Family Heart Association
Wesley House, 7 High Street, Kidlington, Oxford OX5 2DH
Tel: 01865 370292   Website: www.familyheart.org

The Grown Up Congenital Heart (GUCH) Association
12 Rectory Road, Stanford-le-Hope, Essex SS17 0DL
Helpline: 0800 854 759 Fax: 01375 676900
Website: www.guch.demon.co.uk   E-mail: info@guch.demon.co.uk

Heartbeat
This is a voluntary organisation with local branches throughout Britain.
It runs rehabilitation groups using exercise, relaxation and diet, and
invites speakers to monthly meetings. There are opportunities to meet
other heart patients and share concerns and experiences. There will be
a local telephone number available from the cardiac department of your
local hospital.

The Hypertrophic Cardiomyopathy Association
40 The Metro Centre, Tolpits Lane, Watford, Hertfordshire WD1 8SB
Tel: 01923 249977

The Marfan Association
6 Queens Road, Farnborough, Hampshire, GU14 6DH
Tel: 01252 547441 (office hours); 01252 617320 (answerphone)

National Transplant News
Tel: 0208 332 2247

Noonan's Syndrome Society
Unit 5, Brindley Business Park, Chaseside Drive, Cannock,
Staffordshire WS11 1GD
Tel: 01922 415500

The Patients' Association
Helpline: 0845 608 4455   Website: www.patientsassociation.com

Quit
Victory House, Tottenham Court Road, London W1P 0HA
Offers advice on quitting smoking.

Roche Diagnostics
Tel: 01273 480444   Customer Services: 08081 0099 98
Website: www.roche.com
Produces coagucheck S, a patient-orientated device to measure the INR
(which controls the level of Warfarin dosage).

The United Kingdom Council for Psychotherapy
167–169 Great Portland Street, London W1W 5FP
Tel: 0207 436 3002   Fax: 0207 436 3013
E-mail: Ukcp@psychotherapy.org.uk   www.psychotherapy.org.uk

Websites

Websites can give a lot of information – sometimes too much and it can
be worrying. If you find information on a website that concerns you,
make sure that you find time to ask someone who knows more about it
rather than just making yourself anxious.

General

The British Heart Foundation: www.bhf.org.uk

The Family Heart Association: www.familyheart.org
This is patient run and patient orientated.

www.health.havard.edu
Harvard Health letter. A good source of information where précis of new
research can be found.

The Patients' Association: patientsassociation.com

www.wellcome.ac.uk/healthinfo/
Offers health information.

The University of York NHS Centre for Reviews and Dissemination: www.york.ac.uk/inst/crd

Blood Pressure

The Blood Pressure Association: www.bpassoc.org.uk

www.bloodpressure.com
This is a very comprehensive site that answers questions from the basics to the more complex. There is a detailed appendix covering the prescription of tablets. Since this is an American site some of the manufacturers' brand names may be different from those used in the UK. Compare with the UK drug information pharmacists' group website at www.ukdipg.org.uk.

www.hyp.ac.uk/bhs/index.htm
This is a UK website. It is more orientated to the medical profession than the patient, nevertheless it does have information for patients on high blood pressure and its management.

www.successwithchf.com
A very good website that lists the sodium content of common foods.

Cardiac Catheterisation

www.uscuh.com/tour/quicktime/cardiac/cardiac-main.html
This gives you a 3-D virtual reality tour of a cardiac catherterisation.

www.northmemorialcom/nmhc/services/heart/animate.htm
This site includes Quicktime movies about having an angioplasty.

Cardiomyopathy

The UK Cardiomyopathy Organisation: www.cardiomyopathy.org

Complementary Therapies

The Centre for Complementary Health Studies: www.ex.ac.uk/chs

Department of Complementary Medicine:
www.ex.ac.uk/pgms/comphome.htm

Information on unusual complementary treatments:
www.quackwatch.com

Acupuncture

British Acupuncture Council: www.acupuncture.org.uk/

British Medical Acupuncture Society: www.medical-acupuncture.co.uk

International acupuncture associations:
directory.google.com/Top/Health/Alternative/Acupuncture_and
Chinese Medicine/ProfessionalOrganisations/

Herbal Medicine

The American Botanical Council: www.herbalgram.org/

Herbal medicine (Phytonet): www.exeter.ac.uk/phytonet/

Homoeopathy

The Homoeopathic Trust: www.trusthomeopathy.org/

The National Center for Homeopathy in the US: www.homeopathic.org

Hypnosis

The British Society for Medical and Dental Hypnosis: www.bsmdh.org/

The US Society for Clinical and Experimental Hypnosis at:
sunsite.utk.edu/ijceh/scehfram.htm

Massage

American massage therapy: www.amtamassage.org/

Osteopathy

Osteopathic information service: www.osteopathy.org.uk/

Congential Heart Disease

GUCH (Grown Up Congenital Heart Association):
www.guch@demon.co.uk

www.pediheart.org
Includes sections for children and adults concerning congenital heart
disease – excellent website.

www.rch.inimel.edu.au/cardiology/website/index.html
Very good question and answer site for congenital heart disease.

Coronary Heart Disease

www.medcal.co.uk

www.healthpro.org.uk

www.theheart.org (mainly for doctors)

Driving

Advice on conditions forbidding you to drive:
www.open.gov.uk/dvla/dmed1.htm#5

www.fortunecity.co.uk/southbank/hornton/11/hottpic/drive.htm

Exercise

Exercise on prescription: www.doh.gov.uk/exercisereferrals

Heart Failure

www.geocities.com/Heartland/Hills/2571
This is a very good guide to heart failure written by a patient. It is a fantastic source of information and covers many topics including recipes for a reduced-salt diet. Changes in lifestyle are based on real individuals sharing experiences. There is also a comprehensive list of heart drugs (with links covering every aspect, including extracts from journals on recent trials). This site has had more than 3 million hits in the last year.

www.heartfailure.org

www.cardiacfailure.org
These two websites are not nearly as comprehensive as the Heartland site above.

www.successwithchf.com
Contains information on salt intake.

INDEX